EIGHTH EDITION

# PULMONARY PATHOPHYSIOLOGY

THE ESSENTIALS

EIGHTH EDITION

# PULMONARY PATHOPHYSIOLOGY

## THE ESSENTIALS

### John B. West, M.D., Ph.D., D.Sc.

Professor of Medicine and Physiology
University of California, San Diego
School of Medicine
La Jolla, California

Wolters Kluwer | Lippincott Williams & Wilkins
Health
Philadelphia · Baltimore · New York · London
Buenos Aires · Hong Kong · Sydney · Tokyo

*Acquisitions Editor*: Crystal Taylor
*Product Manager*: Catherine Noonan
*Marketing Manager*: Joy Fisher-Williams
*Vendor Manager*: Bridgett Dougherty
*Manufacturing Manager*: Margie Orzech
*Designer*: Holly Mclaughlin
*Compositor*: SPi Global

Eighth Edition

Printed in China

**Copyright © 2013 Lippincott Williams & Wilkins, a Wolters Kluwer business**

351 West Camden Street
Baltimore, MD 21201

Two Commerce Square
2001 Market Street
Philadelphia, PA 19103

First Edition, 1977
Second Edition, 1982
Third Edition, 1987
Fourth Edition, 1992
Fifth Edition, 1998
Sixth Edition, 2003
Seventh Edition, 2008

**Library of Congress Cataloging-in-Publication Data**
West, John B. (John Burnard) Pulmonary pathophysiology : the essentials / John B. West. — 8th ed.
    p. ; cm.
  Companion v. to: Respiratory physiology / John B. Best. 9th ed. c2012.
  Includes bibliographical references and index.
  ISBN 978-1-4511-0713-5
  1. Lungs—Pathophysiology. 2. Pulmonary function tests. I. West, John B. (John Burnard). Respiratory physiology.
II. Title.
  [DNLM: 1. Lung Diseases—physiopathology. 2. Lung—pathology. 3. Respiratory Function Tests. WF 600]
  RC711.W469 2012
  616.2'407—dc23

                                                                              2011028220

To purchase additional copies of this book, call our customer service department at (800) 638-3030 or fax orders to (301) 223-2320. International customers should call (301) 223-2300.

Visit Lippincott Williams & Wilkins on the Internet: http://www.lww.com. Lippincott Williams & Wilkins customer service representatives are available from 8:30 am to 6:00 PM, EST.

CCS0213

To R.B.W.

# Reviewers

Mausam R. Damani, MD
Resident Physician
University of Pennsylvania
Philadelphia, Pennsylvania

Anthony DeAngelis
University of Toledo College of Medicine
Class of 2012
Toledo, Ohio

Andrew J. Degnan
The George Washington University School of Medicine
Class of 2012
Washington, DC

John P. Geibel, MD, DSc
Professor
Department of Surgery
Department of Cellular and Molecular Physiology
Director of Surgical Research
Yale University
New Haven, Connecticut

Michelle Walter
Bastyr University
Class of 2012
Seattle, Washington

# Preface

This book is a companion to *Respiratory Physiology: The Essentials*, 9th edition (Lippincott Williams & Wilkins, 2012), and is about the function of the diseased lung as opposed to the normal lung. It is intended primarily for medical students in their second and subsequent years. However, a concise, amply illustrated account of respiratory function in disease will prove useful to the increasingly large number of physicians (such as anesthesiologists and cardiologists) and other medical personnel (including intensive care nurses and respiratory therapists) who come into contact with respiratory patients. In addition, postgraduate students will find this brief account valuable for reviewing material before examinations.

Many medical schools are constantly trying to emphasize the relevance of the basic science of the first two years to the practice of medicine. Respiratory function can be a model for this. A discussion of a patient with asthma, for example, can quickly and painlessly cover the basic physiology of the airways, blood gases, and lung volumes. I hope that this little book will be helpful in such a course that bridges the preclinical and clinical disciplines.

This book emphasizes the relations between structure and function in the diseased lung. Indeed, readers will find more anatomic pathology than might be expected in a book about pathophysiology. However, function cannot be understood properly without knowledge of structure. It is assumed that students who read this book are also exposed to teaching in pathology.

For this eighth edition, the text has been thoroughly revised and brought up to date in a number of areas including exercise testing, control of ventilation, pathogenesis of asthma, and bronchoactive drugs. However, the length of the book has been kept almost the same in sympathy with the plight of modern medical students.

Other changes improve the didactic nature of the book. All the questions are now in the USMLE format, lists of key concepts have been added at the end of each chapter, and important points are highlighted. In addition there is a brief discussion of the answers to the questions.

I would be grateful for any comments on the selection of material and any factual errors, and I respond to all emails on these subjects.

*John B. West*
jwest@ucsd.edu

# Contents

# Lung Function Tests and What They Mean

We learn how diseased lungs work by doing pulmonary function tests. Accordingly, Part One is devoted to a description of the most important tests and their interpretation. It is assumed that the reader is familiar with the basic physiology of the lung as contained in the companion volume, West JB. *Respiratory Physiology: The Essentials*, 9th ed. Baltimore, MD: Lippincott Williams & Wilkins, 2012.

# Ventilation

The simplest test of lung function is a forced expiration. It is also one of the most informative tests and it requires minimal equipment and trivial calculations. The majority of patients with lung disease have an abnormal forced expiration volume and, very often, the information obtained from this test is useful in their management. In spite of this, the test is not used as often as it should be. For example, it can be valuable in detecting early airway disease, an extremely common and important condition. This chapter also discusses a simple test of uneven ventilation.

## ► Tests of Ventilatory Capacity

### Forced Expiratory Volume

The *forced expiratory volume* (FEV) is the volume of gas exhaled in *1 second* by a forced expiration from full inspiration. The *vital capacity* is the *total* volume of gas that can be exhaled after a full inspiration.

A simple way of making these measurements is shown in Figure 1-1. The patient is comfortably seated in front of a spirometer having a low resistance. He or she breathes in maximally and then exhales as hard and as far as possible. As the spirometer bell moves up, the kymograph pen moves down, thus indicating the expired volume against time.

Figure 1-2A shows a normal tracing. The volume exhaled in 1 second was 4.0 liters and the total volume exhaled was 5.0 liters. These two volumes are therefore the forced expiratory volume in 1 second ($FEV_1$) and the vital capacity. The vital capacity measured with a forced expiration may be less than that measured with a slower exhalation, so that the term *forced vital capacity* (FVC) is generally used. Note that the normal ratio of $FEV_1$ to FVC is approximately 80% but it decreases with age (see Appendix A for normal values).

The FEV can be measured over other times, such as 2 or 3 seconds, but the 1-second value is the most informative. When the subscript is omitted, the time is 1 second.

Figure 1-2B shows the type of tracing obtained from a patient with chronic obstructive pulmonary disease (COPD). Note that the rate at which the air was exhaled was much slower, so that only 1.3 liters were blown out in the first second. In addition, the total volume exhaled was only 3.1 liters. $FEV_1$/FVC was reduced to 42%. These figures are typical of an *obstructive* pattern.

Contrast this pattern with that of Figure 1-2C, which shows the type of tracing obtained from a patient with pulmonary fibrosis. Here, the vital capacity was reduced to 3.1 liters, but a large percentage (90%) was exhaled in the first second. These figures mean *restrictive* disease.

The simple water-filled spirometer shown in Figure 1-1 is now seldom used and has been replaced by electronic spirometers, which often provide a graph to be filed with the patient's chart.

The patient should loosen tight clothing and the mouthpiece should be at a convenient height. One accepted procedure is to allow two practice blows and then record three good test breaths. The highest $FEV_1$ and FVC from these three breaths are then used. The volumes should be converted to body temperature and pressure (see Appendix A).

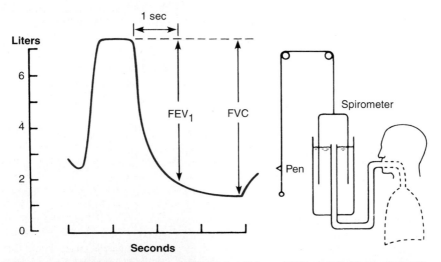

**Figure 1-1. Measurement of Forced Expiratory Volume ($FEV_1$) and Vital Capacity (FVC).**

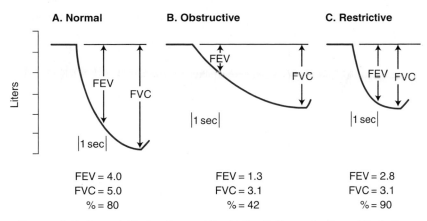

FEV = 4.0
FVC = 5.0
% = 80

FEV = 1.3
FVC = 3.1
% = 42

FEV = 2.8
FVC = 3.1
% = 90

**Figure 1-2.** Normal, Obstructive, and Restrictive Patterns of a Forced Expiration.

The test is often valuable in assessing the efficacy of bronchodilator drugs. If reversible airway obstruction is suspected, the test should be carried out before and after administering the drug (e.g., 0.5% albuterol by nebulizer for 3 minutes). Both the $FEV_1$ and FVC usually increase in a patient with bronchospasm.

## FEV₁ and FVC

The one-second forced expiratory volume together with the forced vital capacity is

a simple test.

often informative.

abnormal in many patients with lung disease.

often valuable in assessing the progress of disease.

## Forced Expiratory Flow

This index is calculated from a forced expiration, as shown in Figure 1-3. The middle half (by volume) of the total expiration is marked and its duration is measured. The $FEF_{25-75\%}$ is the volume in liters divided by the time in seconds.

The correlation between $FEF_{25-75\%}$ and $FEV_1$ is generally close in patients with obstructive pulmonary disease. The changes in $FEF_{25-75\%}$ are often more striking, but the range of normal values is greater.

## Interpretation of Tests of Forced Expiration

In some respects, the lungs and thorax can be regarded as a simple air pump (Figure 1-4). The output of such a pump depends on the stroke volume, the resistance of the airways, and the force applied to the piston. The last factor is relatively unimportant in a forced expiration, as we shall presently see.

The *vital capacity* (or forced vital capacity) is a measure of the stroke volume, and any reduction of it affects the ventilatory capacity. Causes of stroke volume reduction include diseases of the thoracic cage, such as kyphoscoliosis, ankylosing spondylitis, and acute injuries; diseases affecting the nerve supply to the respiratory muscles or the muscles themselves, such as poliomyelitis and muscular dystrophy; abnormalities of the pleural cavity, such as pneumothorax and pleural thickening; disease in the lung itself, such as fibrosis, which reduces

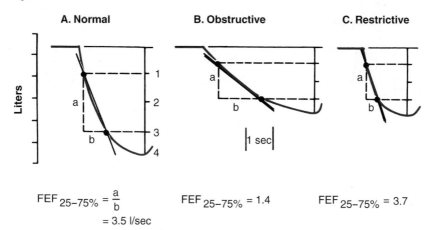

$$\text{FEF}_{25-75\%} = \frac{a}{b}$$
$$= 3.5 \text{ l/sec}$$

$$\text{FEF}_{25-75\%} = 1.4$$

$$\text{FEF}_{25-75\%} = 3.7$$

**Figure 1-3.** Calculation of Forced Expiratory Flow (FEF$_{25-75\%}$) from a Forced Expiration.

its distensibility; space-occupying lesions, such as cysts; or an increased pulmonary blood volume, as in left heart failure. In addition, there are diseases of the airways that cause them to close prematurely during expiration, thus limiting the volume that can be exhaled. This occurs in asthma and bronchitis.

The *forced expiratory volume* (and related indices such as the FEF$_{25-75\%}$) is affected by the airway resistance during forced expiration. Any increase in resistance reduces the ventilatory capacity. Causes include bronchoconstriction, as in asthma or following the inhalation of irritants such as cigarette smoke; structural changes in the airways, as in chronic bronchitis; obstructions within the airways, such as an inhaled foreign body or excess bronchial secretions; and destructive processes in the lung parenchyma, which interfere with the radial traction that normally holds the airways open.

The simple model of Figure 1-4 introduces the factors limiting the ventilatory capacity of the diseased lung, but we need to refine the model to obtain a better understanding. For example, the airways are actually *inside*, not *outside*, the pump, as shown in Figure 1-4. Useful additional information comes from the flow-volume curve.

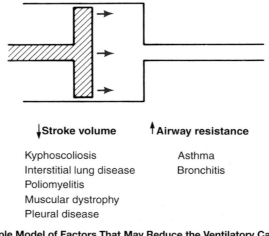

↓Stroke volume        ↑Airway resistance

Kyphoscoliosis              Asthma
Interstitial lung disease   Bronchitis
Poliomyelitis
Muscular dystrophy
Pleural disease

**Figure 1-4. Simple Model of Factors That May Reduce the Ventilatory Capacity.** The stroke volume may be reduced by diseases of the chest wall, lung parenchyma, respiratory muscles, and pleura. Airway resistance is increased in asthma and bronchitis.

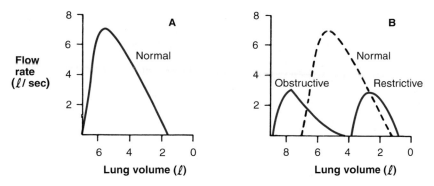

**Figure 1-5. Expiratory Flow-Volume Curves. A.** Normal. **B.** Obstructive and restrictive patterns.

## Expiratory Flow-Volume Curve

If we record flow rate and volume during a maximal forced expiration, we obtain a pattern like that shown in Figure 1-5A. A curious feature of the flow-volume curve is that it is virtually impossible to get outside it. For example, if we begin by exhaling slowly and then exert maximum effort, the flow rate increases to the envelope but not beyond. Clearly, something very powerful is limiting the maximum flow rate at a given volume. This factor is *dynamic compression of the airways*.

Figure 1-5B shows typical patterns found in obstructive and restrictive lung disease. In obstructive diseases, such as chronic bronchitis and emphysema, the maximal expiration typically begins and ends at abnormally high lung volumes, and the flow rates are much lower than normal. In addition, the curve may have a scooped-out appearance. By contrast, patients with restrictive disease, such as interstitial fibrosis, operate at low lung volumes. Their flow envelope is flattened compared with a normal curve, but if flow rate is related to lung volume, the flow is seen to be higher than normal (Figure 1-5B). Note that the figure shows absolute lung volumes, although these cannot be obtained from a forced expiration. They require an additional measurement of residual volume.

To understand these patterns, consider the pressures inside and outside the airways (Figure 1-6) (see *Respiratory Physiology: The Essentials*, 9th ed., p. 121). Before inspiration (A), the pressures in the mouth, airways, and alveoli are all atmospheric because there is no flow. Intrapleural pressure is, say, 5 cm $H_2O$ below atmospheric pressure, and we assume that the same pressure exists outside the airways (although this is an oversimplification). Thus, the pressure difference expanding the airways is 5 cm $H_2O$. At the beginning of inspiration (B), all pressures fall and the pressure difference holding the airways open increases to 6 cm $H_2O$. At the end of inspiration (C), this pressure is 8 cm $H_2O$.

### Dynamic Compression of the Airways

limits flow rate during a forced expiration.

causes flow to be independent of effort.

may limit flow during normal expiration in some patients with COPD.

is a major factor limiting exercise in COPD.

Early in a forced expiration (D), both intrapleural and alveolar pressures rise greatly. The pressure at some point in the airways increases, but not as much as alveolar pressure because

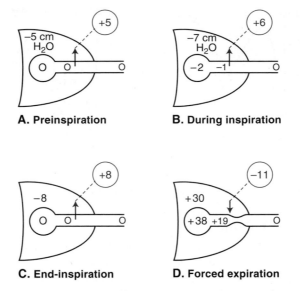

**A. Preinspiration**    **B. During inspiration**

**C. End-inspiration**    **D. Forced expiration**

**Figure 1-6.** Diagram to Explain Dynamic Compression of the Airways during a Forced Expiration (see text for details).

of the pressure drop caused by flow. Under these circumstances, we have a pressure difference of 11 cm $H_2O$, which tends to *close* the airways. Airway compression occurs, and now flow is determined by the difference between alveolar pressure and the pressure outside the airways at the collapse point (Starling resistor effect). Note that this pressure difference (8 cm $H_2O$ in D) is the static recoil pressure of the lung and it depends only on lung volume and compliance. It is *independent* of expiratory effort.

How then can we explain the abnormal patterns in Figure 1-5B? In the patient with chronic bronchitis and emphysema, the low flow rate in relation to lung volume is caused by several factors. There may be thickening of the walls of the airways and excessive secretions in the lumen because of bronchitis; both increase the flow resistance. The number of small airways may be reduced because of destruction of lung tissue. Also, the patient may have a reduced static recoil pressure (even though lung volume is greatly increased) because of breakdown of elastic alveolar walls. Finally, the normal support offered to the airways by the traction of the surrounding parenchyma is probably impaired because of loss of alveolar walls, and the airways therefore collapse more easily than they should. These factors are considered in more detail in Chapter 4.

The patient with interstitial fibrosis has normal (or high) flow rates in relation to lung volume because the lung static recoil pressures are high and the caliber of the airways may be normal (or even increased) at a given lung volume. However, because of the greatly reduced compliance of the lung, volumes are very small, and absolute flow rates are therefore reduced. These changes are further discussed in Chapter 5.

This analysis shows that Figure 1-4 is a considerable oversimplification and that the forced expiratory volume, which seems so straightforward at first, is affected both by the airways and by the lung parenchyma. Thus, the terms "obstructive" and "restrictive" conceal a good deal of pathophysiology.

## Partitioning of Flow Resistance from the Flow-Volume Curve

When the airways collapse during a forced expiration, the flow rate is determined by the resistance of the airways up to the point of collapse (Figure 1-7). Beyond this point, the

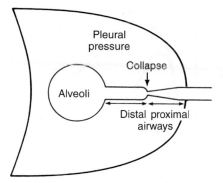

**Figure 1-7. Dynamic Compression of the Airways.** When this occurs during a forced expiration, only the resistance of the airways distal to the point of collapse (upstream segment) determines the flow rate. In the last stages of a forced vital capacity test, only the peripheral small airways are distal to the collapsed point and therefore determine the flow.

resistance of the airways is immaterial. Collapse occurs at (or near) the point where the pressure inside the airways is equal to the intrapleural pressure (*equal pressure point*). This is believed to be in the vicinity of the lobar bronchi early in a forced expiration. However, as lung volume reduces and the airways narrow, their resistance increases. As a result, pressure is lost more rapidly and the collapse point moves into more distal airways. Thus, late in forced expiration, flow is increasingly determined by the properties of the small distal peripheral airways.

These peripheral airways (say, less than 2 mm in diameter) normally contribute less than 20% of the total airway resistance. Therefore, changes in them are difficult to detect and they constitute a "silent zone." However, it is likely that some of the earliest changes in COPD occur in these small airways, and therefore maximum flow rate late in a forced expiration is often taken to reflect peripheral airway resistance.

## Maximum Flows from the Flow-Volume Curve

Maximum flow ($\dot{V}$max) is frequently measured after 50% ($\dot{V}$max$_{50\%}$) or 75% ($\dot{V}$max$_{75\%}$) of the vital capacity has been exhaled. Figure 1-8 shows the abnormal flow pattern typically seen in tests of patients with COPD. The later in expiration that the flow is measured, the more the measurement reflects the resistance of the very small airways. Some studies have shown abnormalities in the $\dot{V}$max$_{75\%}$ when other indices of a forced expiration, such as the $FEV_1$ or $FEF_{25-75\%}$, were normal.

## Peak Expiratory Flow Rate

Peak expiratory flow rate is the maximum flow rate during a forced expiration starting from total lung capacity. It can be conveniently estimated with an inexpensive, portable peak flow meter. The measurement is not precise and it depends on the patient's effort. Nevertheless, it is a valuable tool for following disease, especially asthma, and the patient can easily make repeated measurements in the home or workplace and keep a log to show to the physician.

## Inspiratory Flow-Volume Curve

The flow-volume curve is also often measured during inspiration. This curve is not affected by the dynamic compression of the airways because the pressures during inspiration always

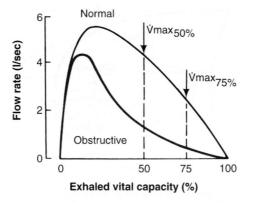

**Figure 1-8. Example of an Expiratory Flow-Volume Curve in COPD.** Note the scooped-out appearance. The *arrows* show the maximum expiratory flow after 50% and 75% of the vital capacity have been exhaled.

expand the bronchi (Figure 1-6). However, the curve is useful in detecting upper airway obstruction, which flattens the curve because maximum flow is limited (Figure 1-9). Causes include glottic and tracheal stenosis and tracheal narrowing as a result of a compressing neoplasm. The expiratory flow-volume curve is also flattened by fixed (nonvariable) upper airway obstruction.

## ▶ Tests of Uneven Ventilation

### Single-Breath Nitrogen Test
The tests described so far measure ventilatory capacity. The single-breath nitrogen test measures inequality of ventilation. This topic is somewhat different but is conveniently described here.

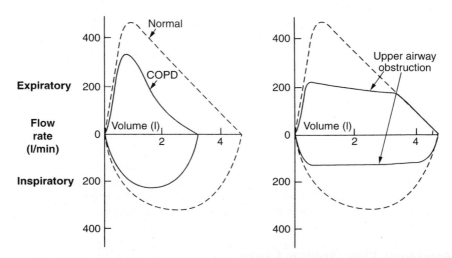

**Figure 1-9. Expiratory and Inspiratory Flow-Volume Curves.** In normal subjects and patients with COPD, inspiratory flow rates are normal (or nearly so). In fixed upper airway obstruction, both inspiratory and expiratory flow rates are reduced.

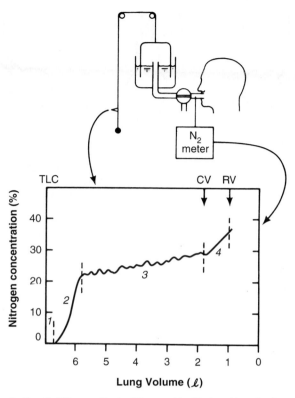

**Figure 1-10. Single-Breath Nitrogen Test of Uneven Ventilation.** Note the four phases of the expired tracing. *TLC*, total lung capacity; *CV*, closing volume; *RV*, residual volume.

Suppose a patient takes a vital capacity inspiration of oxygen, that is, to total lung capacity, and then exhales slowly as far as he can, that is, to residual volume. If we measure the nitrogen concentration at the mouthpiece with a rapid nitrogen analyzer, we record a pattern as shown in Figure 1-10. Four phases can be recognized. In the first, which is very short, pure oxygen is exhaled from the upper airways and the nitrogen concentration is zero. In the second phase, the nitrogen concentration rises rapidly as the anatomic dead space is washed out by alveolar gas. This phase is also short.

The third phase consists of alveolar gas, and the tracing is nearly flat with a small upward slope in normal subjects. This portion is often known as the alveolar plateau. In patients with uneven ventilation, the third phase is steeper, and the slope is a measure of the inequality of ventilation. It is expressed as the percentage increase in nitrogen concentration per liter of expired volume. In carrying out this test, the expiratory flow rate should be no more than 0.5 liters/s in order to reduce the variability of the results.

The reason for the rise in nitrogen concentration in phase 4 is that some regions of lung are poorly ventilated and therefore receive relatively little of the breath of oxygen. These areas therefore have a relatively high concentration of nitrogen because there is less oxygen to dilute this gas. Also, these poorly ventilated regions tend to empty last.

Three possible mechanisms of uneven ventilation are shown in Figure 1-11. In A, the region is poorly ventilated because of partial obstruction of its airway, and because of this high resistance, the region empties late. In fact, the rate of emptying of such a region is determined by its time constant, which is given by the product of its airway resistance (R)

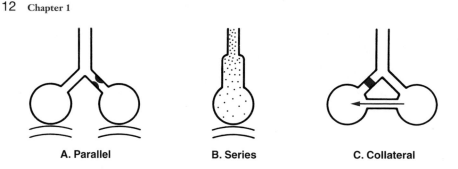

**Figure 1-11. Three Mechanisms of Uneven Ventilation.** In parallel inequality (**A**), flow to regions with long time constants is reduced. In series inequality (**B**), dilation of a small airway may result in incomplete diffusion along a terminal lung unit. Collateral ventilation (**C**) may also cause series inequality.

and compliance (C). The larger the time constant (RC), the longer it takes to empty. This mechanism is known as *parallel* inequality of ventilation.

Figure 1-11B shows the mechanism known as *series* inequality. Here there is a dilation of peripheral airspaces, which causes differences of ventilation *along* the air passages of a lung unit. In this context, we should recall that inspired gas reaches the terminal bronchioles by convective flow, that is, like water running through a hose, but its subsequent movement to the alveoli is chiefly accomplished by diffusion within the airways. Normally, the distances are so short that nearly complete equilibration of gas concentrations is established quickly. However, if the small airways enlarge, as occurs, for example, in centriacinar emphysema (see Figure 4-4), the concentration of inspired gas in the most distal airways may remain low. Again, these poorly ventilated regions empty last.

Figure 1-11C shows another form of series inequality that occurs when some lung units receive their inspired gas from neighboring units rather than from the large airways. This is known as collateral ventilation and appears to be an important process in COPD and asthma.

## Uneven Ventilation

occurs in many patients with lung disease.

is an important factor contributing to impaired gas exchange.

is conveniently measured with the single-breath $N_2$ test.

There is still uncertainty about the relative importance of parallel and series inequality. It is likely that both operate to a small extent in people with normal ventilation and to a much greater degree in patients with obstructive pulmonary disease. Whatever the mechanism, the single-breath nitrogen test is a simple, rapid, and reliable way of measuring the degree of uneven ventilation in the lung. This is increased in most obstructive and many restrictive types of lung disease (see Chapters 4 and 5).

## Closing Volume

Toward the end of the vital capacity expiration shown in Figure 1-10, the nitrogen concentration rises abruptly, signaling the onset of airway closure, or phase 4. The lung volume at which phase 4 begins is called the *closing volume*, and the closing volume plus the residual volume is known as the *closing capacity*. In practice, the onset of phase 4 is obtained by drawing a straight line through the alveolar plateau (phase 3) and noting the last point of departure of the nitrogen tracing from this line.

Unfortunately, the junction between phases 3 and 4 is seldom as clear-cut as in Figure 1-10, and there is considerable variation of this volume when the test is repeated by a patient. The test is most useful in the presence of small amounts of disease because severe disease distorts the tracing so much that the closing volume cannot be identified.

The mechanism of the onset of phase 4 is still uncertain, but is believed to be closure of small airways in the lowest part of the lung. At residual volume just before the single breath of oxygen is inhaled, the nitrogen concentration is virtually uniform throughout the lung, but the basal alveoli are much smaller than the apical alveoli in the upright subject because of distortion of the lung by its weight. Indeed, the lowest portions are compressed so much that the small airways in the region of the respiratory bronchioles are closed. However, at the end of a vital capacity inspiration, all the alveoli are approximately the same size. Thus, the nitrogen at the base is diluted much more than that of the apex by the breath of oxygen.

During the subsequent expiration, the upper and lower zones empty together and the expired nitrogen concentration is nearly constant (Figure 1-10). As soon as dependent airways begin to close, however, the higher nitrogen concentration in the upper zones preferentially affects the expired concentration, causing an abrupt rise. Moreover, as airway closure proceeds up the lung, the expired nitrogen progressively increases.

Some studies show that in some subjects the closing volume is the same in the weightlessness of space as in normal gravity. This finding suggests that compression of a dependent lung is not always the mechanism.

The volume at which airways close is age dependent, being as low as 10% of the vital capacity in young normal subjects but increasing to 40% (i.e., approximately the FRC) at about the age of 65 years. There is some evidence that the test is sensitive to small amounts of disease. For example, apparently healthy cigarette smokers sometimes have increased closing volumes when their ventilatory capacity is normal.

## Other Tests of Uneven Ventilation

Uneven ventilation can also be measured by a multibreath nitrogen washout during oxygen breathing. Topographic inequality of ventilation can be determined using radioactive xenon. This chapter is confined to single-breath tests; other measurements are referred to in Chapter 3.

## Tests of Early Airway Disease

There has been great interest in the possible use of some tests described in this chapter to identify patients with early airway disease. Once a patient develops the full picture of COPD, the results of treatment are generally disappointing. The hope is that by identifying disease at an early stage, its progression can be slowed, for example, by the patient stopping cigarette smoking.

Among the tests that have been examined in this context are the $FEV_1$, $FEF_{25-75\%}$, $\dot{V}max_{50\%}$ and $\dot{V}max_{75\%}$, and the closing volume. Assessment of these tests is difficult because it depends on prospective studies and large control groups. It is now clear that the original test of $FEV_1$ remains one of the most reliable and valuable tests. While more sophisticated tests should be investigated, measuring the $FEV_1$ and FVC remains mandatory.

## KEY CONCEPTS

1. The one-second forced expiratory volume and the forced vital capacity are easy tests to do, require little equipment, and are often very informative.

2. Dynamic compression of the airways is common in COPD and is a major case of disability.

3. The small airways (less than 2 mm in diameter) are often the site of early airway disease, but the changes are difficult to detect.

4. Uneven ventilation is common in airway diseases and can be measured with a single-breath $N_2$ test.

5. The closing volume is often increased in mild airway disease and it also increases with age.

## QUESTIONS

For each question, choose the best answer.

1. The one-second forced expiratory volume test

    A. Is difficult to perform.
    B. Can be used to assess the efficacy of bronchodilators.
    C. Is unaffected by dynamic compression of the airways.
    D. Is reduced in patients with fibrosis but not COPD.
    E. Increases with age.

2. Maximum flow rate during most of a forced expiration is limited by

    A. Turbulence in the trachea.
    B. Action of the diaphragm.
    C. Contraction of the intercostal muscles.
    D. Power of the abdominal muscles.
    E. Compression of the airways.

3. The $FEV_1$ in a patient with COPD is reduced by

    A. Increased lung compliance.
    B. Increase in the number of small airways.
    C. Increased radial traction on the airways.
    D. Increased elastic recoil of the lung.
    E. Hypertrophy of the diaphragm.

4. The $FEV_1$ and FVC are measured in a patient with interstitial fibrosis of the lung. We expect

    A. Increased $FEV_1$.
    B. Increased FVC.
    C. Increased $FEV_1/FVC$.
    D. Decreased expiratory flow rate when related to lung volume.
    E. Abnormally high flow rate early in expiration.

5. The inspiratory flow-volume curve is most valuable for

    A. Detecting fixed upper airway obstruction.
    B. Measuring the response to bronchodilator drugs.
    C. Differentiating between chronic bronchitis and emphysema.
    D. Detecting resistance in small peripheral airways.
    E. Detecting fatigue of the diaphragm.

6. Concerning the single-breath nitrogen test,

    A. It is usually normal in mild COPD.
    B. The slope of phase 3 is increased in chronic bronchitis.
    C. In phase 3, well-ventilated units empty last.
    D. In normal subjects, the last expired gas comes from the base of the lung.
    E. The expiratory flow rate should be as fast as possible.

**7.** The closing volume as measured from the single-breath $N_2$ test

    A. Decreases with age.
    B. Is highly reproducible.
    C. Is affected by the small, peripheral airways.
    D. Is most informative in patients with severe lung disease.
    E. Is normal in mild COPD.

# Gas Exchange

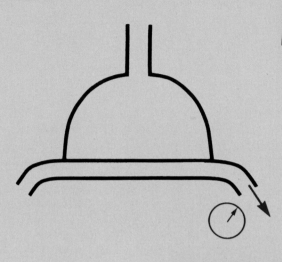

**2**

C hapter 1 dealt with the simplest test of lung function: the forced expiration. In addition, we looked briefly at the single-breath test of uneven ventilation. In this chapter, we turn to the most important measurement in the management of respiratory failure: arterial blood gases. Another test of gas exchange, the diffusing capacity, is also discussed.

## ▶ Blood Gases

### Arterial $P_{O_2}$

#### Measurement

It is often essential to know the partial pressure of oxygen in the arterial blood of acutely ill patients. With modern blood gas electrodes, the measurement of arterial $P_{O_2}$ is relatively simple, and the test is mandatory in the management of patients with respiratory failure.

Arterial blood is usually taken by puncturing the radial artery or from an indwelling radial artery catheter. The $P_{O_2}$ is measured by the polarographic principle, that is, the test measures the current that flows when a small voltage is applied to electrodes.

#### Normal Values

The normal value for $P_{O_2}$ in young adults averages approximately 95 mm Hg, with a range of approximately 85 to 100 mm Hg. The normal value decreases steadily with age, and the average is approximately 85 mm Hg at age 60 years. The cause of the fall in $P_{O_2}$ with age is probably increasing ventilation–perfusion inequality (see the section later in this chapter).

Whenever we read a report of an arterial $P_{O_2}$ test, we should have the oxygen dissociation curve at the back of our minds. Figure 2-1 reminds us of two anchor points on the normal curve. One is arterial blood ($P_{O_2}$, 100; $O_2$ saturation, 97%) and the other is mixed venous blood ($P_{O_2}$, 40; $O_2$ saturation, 75%). Also we should recall that above 60 mm Hg, the $O_2$ saturation exceeds 90% and the curve is fairly flat. The curve is shifted to the right by an increase in temperature, $P_{CO_2}$, and $H^+$ concentration (these all occur in exercising muscle when enhanced unloading of $O_2$ is advantageous). The curve is also shifted to the right by an increase in 2,3-diphosphoglycerate (DPG) inside the red cells. 2,3-DPG is depleted in stored blood but is increased in prolonged hypoxia.

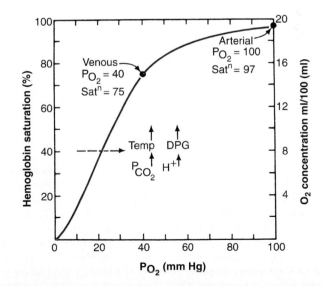

**Figure 2-1. Anchor Points of the Oxygen Dissociation Curve.** The curve is shifted to the right by an increase in temperature, $P_{CO_2}$, $H^+$, and 2,3-DPG. The oxygen concentration scale is based on a hemoglobin concentration of 14.5 g/100 ml.

## Causes of Hypoxemia

There are four primary causes of a reduced $P_{O_2}$ in arterial blood:

**1.** Hypoventilation

**2.** Diffusion impairment

**3.** Shunt

**4.** Ventilation–perfusion inequality

A fifth cause, reduction of inspired $P_{O_2}$, is seen only in special circumstances such as at high altitude or when breathing a gas mixture of low oxygen concentration.

### Hypoventilation

This means that the volume of fresh gas going to the alveoli per unit time (alveolar ventilation) is reduced. If the resting oxygen consumption is not correspondingly reduced, hypoxemia inevitably results. Hypoventilation is commonly caused by diseases outside the lungs; indeed, very often the lungs are normal.

Two cardinal physiologic features of hypoventilation should be emphasized. First, it *always* causes a rise in $P_{CO_2}$ and this is a valuable diagnostic feature. The relationship between the arterial $P_{CO_2}$ and the level of alveolar ventilation in the normal lung is a simple one and is given by the *alveolar ventilation equation*:

$$P_{CO_2} = \frac{\dot{V}_{CO_2}}{\dot{V}_A} \cdot K, \qquad \text{(Eq. 2.1)}$$

where $\dot{V}_{CO_2}$ is the $CO_2$ output, $\dot{V}_A$ is the alveolar ventilation, and K is a constant (see Appendix A for a list of symbols). This means that if the alveolar ventilation is halved, the $P_{CO_2}$ is doubled. If the patient does not have a raised arterial $P_{CO_2}$, he or she is not hypoventilating!

Second, the hypoxemia can be abolished easily by increasing the inspired $P_{O_2}$ by delivering oxygen via a face mask. This can be seen from the *alveolar gas equation*:

$$P_{A_{O_2}} = P_{I_{O_2}} - \frac{P_{A_{CO_2}}}{R} + F, \qquad \text{(Eq. 2.2)}$$

where F is a small correction factor that can be ignored. We will also assume that the alveolar and arterial $P_{CO_2}$ values are the same. This equation states that if the arterial $P_{CO_2}$ ($P_{A_{CO_2}}$) and respiratory exchange ratio (R) remain constant (they will, if the alveolar ventilation and metabolic rate remain unaltered), every mm Hg rise in inspired $P_{O_2}$ ($P_{I_{O_2}}$) produces a corresponding rise in the alveolar $P_{O_2}$ ($P_{A_{O_2}}$). Because it is easily possible to increase the inspired $P_{O_2}$ by several hundred mm Hg, the hypoxemia of pure hypoventilation can readily be abolished.

It is also important to appreciate that the arterial $P_{O_2}$ cannot fall to very low levels from pure hypoventilation. Referring to Equation 2.2 again, we can see that if R = 1, the alveolar $P_{O_2}$ falls 1 mm Hg for every 1 mm Hg rise in $P_{CO_2}$. This means that severe hypoventilation sufficient to double the $P_{CO_2}$ from 40 to 80 mm Hg only decreases the alveolar $P_{O_2}$ from, say, 100 to 60 mm Hg. If $R = 0.8$, the fall is somewhat greater, say, to 50 mm Hg. Also, the arterial $P_{O_2}$ is usually a few mm Hg lower than the alveolar value. Even so, the arterial $O_2$ saturation will be near 80% (Figure 2-2). However, this is a severe degree of $CO_2$ retention that may result in substantial respiratory acidosis, a pH of around 7.2, and a very sick patient! Thus, hypoxemia is not the dominant feature of hypoventilation.

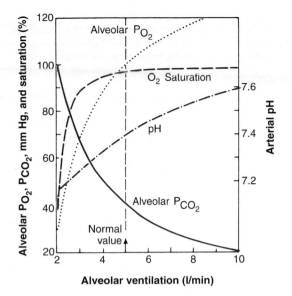

**Figure 2-2. Gas Exchange During Hypoventilation.** Values are approximate.

The causes of hypoventilation are shown in Figure 2-3 and listed in Table 2.1. In addition, hypoventilation is seen in some extremely obese patients who have somnolence, polycythemia, and excessive appetite. This has been dubbed the "pickwickian syndrome" after the fat boy, Joe, in Charles Dickens's *Pickwick Papers*. The cause of the hypoventilation is uncertain, but the increased work of breathing associated with obesity is probably a factor, although some patients appear to have an abnormality of the central nervous system. There is also a rare condition of idiopathic hypoventilation known as Ondine's Curse.

*Sleep apnea.* This can be divided into *central,* where there are no respiratory efforts, and *obstructive,* where, despite activity of the respiratory muscles, there is no airflow.

*Central sleep apnea* often occurs in patients with hypoventilation because respiratory drive is depressed during sleep. During REM sleep, breathing is often irregular and unresponsive to chemical and vagal drives. An exception is hypoxemia, which usually remains a powerful

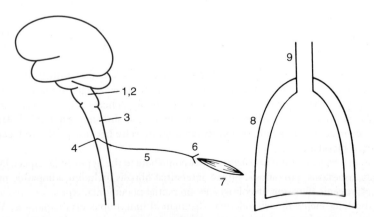

**Figure 2-3. Causes of Hypoventilation.** (See Table 2.1 for details.)

| Table 2.1 | Some Causes of Hypoventilation (see Figure 2-3) |
|---|---|

1. Depression of the respiratory center by drugs (e.g., barbiturates and morphine derivatives)
2. Diseases of the medulla (e.g., encephalitis, hemorrhage, neoplasms [rare])
3. Abnormalities of the spinal cord (e.g., following high dislocation)
4. Anterior horn cell disease (e.g., poliomyelitis)
5. Diseases of the nerves to the respiratory muscles (e.g., in the Guillain-Barré syndrome or diphtheria)
6. Diseases of the myoneural junction (e.g., myasthenia gravis, anticholinesterase poisoning)
7. Diseases of the respiratory muscles (e.g., progressive muscular dystrophy)
8. Thoracic cage abnormalities (e.g., crushed chest)
9. Upper-airway obstruction (e.g., tracheal compression by enlarged lymph nodes)

stimulus to breathe. In Cheyne-Stokes breathing, the tidal volume waxes and wanes, and there are often apneic periods. Periodic breathing is often seen in normal people at high altitude.

*Obstructive sleep apnea* is common. The first reports were in obese patients, but it is now recognized that the condition is not confined to them. Airway obstruction can be caused by backward movement of the tongue, collapse of the pharyngeal walls, greatly enlarged tonsils or adenoids, and other anatomic causes of pharyngeal narrowing. Loud snoring often occurs, and the patient may wake violently after an apneic episode. Chronic sleep deprivation sometimes occurs, and the patient may have daytime somnolence, impaired cognitive function, chronic fatigue, morning headaches, and personality disturbances such as paranoia, hostility, and agitated depression. Treatment by continuous positive airway pressure (CPAP) by means of a face mask during sleep is often effective. This reduces the daytime somnolence and can have other benefits such as reducing systemic hypertension, probably as a result of lowering the blood catecholamine levels, which are elevated by the apneic episodes.

A condition that affects infants is the *sudden infant death syndrome* (SIDS). When this syndrome occurs, the child is found dead typically in the crib with no apparent cause. The cause of this syndrome is still obscure. One hypothesis is that the nervous control of ventilation is not fully developed and the respiratory muscles are poorly coordinated.

*Diffusion Impairment*

This means that equilibration does not occur between the $P_{O_2}$ in the pulmonary capillary blood and alveolar gas. Figure 2-4 reminds us of the time course for $P_{O_2}$ along a pulmonary capillary. Under normal resting conditions, the capillary blood $P_{O_2}$ almost reaches that of alveolar gas after about 1/3 of the total contact time of 3/4 second available in the capillary. Thus, there is plenty of time in reserve. Even with severe exercise, when the contact time may perhaps be reduced to as little as 1/4 second, equilibration almost always occurs.

However, in some diseases, the blood–gas barrier is thickened and diffusion is so slowed that equilibration may be incomplete. Figure 2-5 shows a histologic section of lung from a patient with interstitial fibrosis. Note that the normally delicate alveolar walls are grossly widened. In such a lung, we expect a slower time course, as shown in Figure 2-4. Any hypoxemia that occurred at rest would be exaggerated on exercise because of the reduced contact time between blood and gas.

Diseases in which diffusion impairment may contribute to the hypoxemia, especially on exercise, include asbestosis, sarcoidosis, diffuse interstitial fibrosis including idiopathic pulmonary fibrosis (cryptogenic fibrosing alveolitis) and interstitial pneumonia, connective tissue diseases affecting the lung including scleroderma, rheumatoid lung, lupus erythematosus, Wegener's granulomatosis, Goodpasture's syndrome, and alveolar cell carcinoma. In all these conditions,

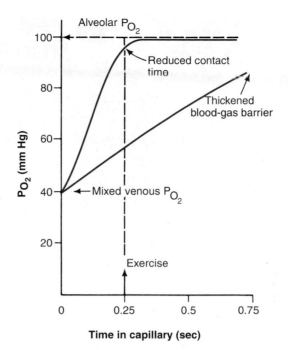

**Figure 2-4. Changes in $P_{O_2}$ Along the Pulmonary Capillary.** During exercise, the time available for $O_2$ diffusion across the blood–gas barrier is reduced. A thickened alveolar wall slows the rate of diffusion.

the diffusion path from alveolar gas to red blood cell may be increased, at least in some regions of the lung, and the time course for oxygenation may be affected, as shown in Figure 2-4.

However, the importance of diffusion impairment to the arterial hypoxemia in these patients is less than it was once thought to be. As has been emphasized, the normal lung has lots of diffusion time in reserve. In addition, if we look at Figure 2-5, it is impossible to believe that the normal relationships between ventilation and blood flow can be preserved in a lung with such an abnormal architecture. We will see shortly that ventilation–perfusion inequality is a powerful cause of hypoxemia, which is undoubtedly operating in these patients. Thus, how much additional hypoxemia should be attributed to diffusion impairment is difficult to know. It is clear that at least some of the hypoxemia on exercise is caused by this mechanism (see Figure 5-6).

Hypoxemia could also result from an extreme reduction in contact time. Suppose that so much blood flow is diverted away from other regions of the lung (e.g., by a large pulmonary embolus) that the time for oxygenation within the capillary is reduced to one-tenth normal. Figure 2-4 shows that hypoxemia would then be inevitable.

Hypoxemia caused by diffusion impairment can be corrected readily by administering 100% oxygen to the patient. The resultant large increase in alveolar $P_{O_2}$ of several hundred mm Hg can easily overcome the increased diffusion resistance of the thickened blood–gas barrier. Carbon dioxide elimination is generally unaffected by diffusion abnormalities. Most patients with the diseases listed earlier do not have carbon dioxide retention. Indeed, typically the arterial $P_{CO_2}$ is slightly lower than normal because ventilation is overstimulated, either by the hypoxemia or by intrapulmonary receptors.

*Shunt*
A shunt allows some blood to reach the arterial system without passing through ventilated regions of the lung. Intrapulmonary shunts can be caused by arterial–venous malformations

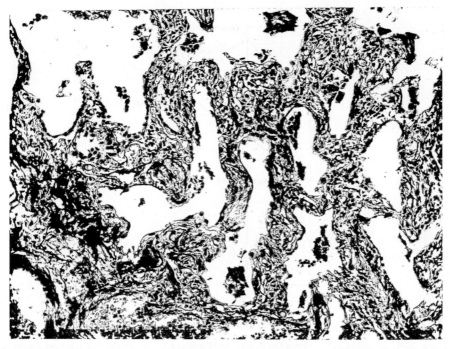

**Figure 2-5. Section of Lung from a Patient with Diffuse Interstitial Fibrosis.** Note the extreme thickening of the alveolar walls, which constitutes a barrier to diffusion (compare with Figures 5-1, 5-3, and 10-5). (From Hinson KFW. Diffuse pulmonary fibrosis. *Hum Pathol* 1970;1:275–288.)

that often have a genetic basis. In addition, an unventilated but perfused area of lung, for example, a consolidated pneumonic lobule, constitutes a shunt. It might be argued that the latter example is simply one extreme of the spectrum of ventilation–perfusion ratios and that it is therefore more reasonable to classify hypoxemia caused by this under the heading of ventilation–perfusion inequality. However, shunt causes such a characteristic pattern of gas exchange during 100% oxygen breathing that it is convenient to include unventilated alveoli under this heading. Very large shunts are often seen in the adult respiratory distress syndrome (see Chapter 8). Many shunts are extrapulmonary, including those that occur in congenital heart disease through atrial or ventricular septal defects or a patent ductus arteriosus. In such patients, there must be a rise in right heart pressure to cause a shunt from right to left.

If a patient with a shunt is given pure oxygen to breathe, the arterial $P_{O_2}$ fails to rise to the level seen in normal subjects. Figure 2-6 shows that although the end-capillary $P_{O_2}$ may be as high as that in alveolar gas, the $O_2$ concentration of the shunted blood is as low as in venous blood if the shunt is mixed venous blood. When a small amount of shunted blood is added to arterial blood, the $O_2$ concentration is depressed. This causes a large fall in arterial $P_{O_2}$ because the $O_2$ dissociation curve is so flat in its upper range. As a result, it is possible to detect small shunts by measuring the arterial $P_{O_2}$ during 100% $O_2$ breathing.

Only shunts behave in this way is a point of practical importance. In the other three causes of hypoxemia (hypoventilation, diffusion impairment, and ventilation–perfusion inequality) the arterial $P_{O_2}$ nearly reaches the normal level seen in healthy subjects during 100% $O_2$ breathing. This may take a long time in some patients who have poorly ventilated alveoli because the nitrogen takes so long to wash out completely that the $P_{O_2}$ is slow to reach its final level. This is probably the reason why the arterial $P_{O_2}$ of patients with chronic obstructive pulmonary disease (COPD) may only rise to 400 to 500 mm Hg after 15 minutes of 100% $O_2$ breathing.

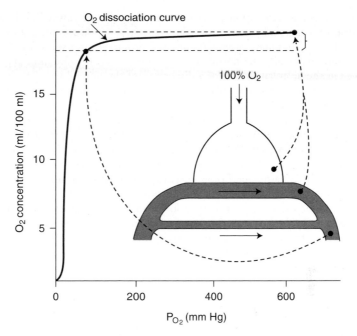

**Figure 2-6. Depression of the Arterial $P_{O_2}$ by a Shunt During 100% $O_2$ Breathing.** The addition of a small amount of shunted blood with its low $O_2$ concentration greatly reduces the $P_{O_2}$ of arterial blood. This is because the $O_2$ dissociation curve is so flat when the $P_{O_2}$ is high.

If the shunt is caused by mixed venous blood, its magnitude during $O_2$ breathing can be determined from the *shunt equation*:

$$\frac{\dot{Q}_S}{\dot{Q}_T} = \frac{C_{C'} - C_a}{C_{C'} - C_{\bar{v}}} \tag{Eq. 2.3}$$

where $\dot{Q}_S$ and $\dot{Q}_T$ refer to the shunt and total blood flows, and $C_{c'}$, $C_a$, and $C_{\bar{v}}$ refer to the $O_2$ concentrations of end-capillary, arterial, and mixed venous blood. The $O_2$ concentration of the end-capillary blood is calculated from the alveolar $P_{O_2}$, assuming complete equilibration between the alveolar gas and the blood. Mixed venous blood is sampled with a catheter in the pulmonary artery. The denominator in Equation 2.3 can also be estimated from the measured oxygen uptake and cardiac output.

Shunt does not usually result in a raised arterial $P_{CO_2}$. The tendency for this to rise is generally countered by the chemoreceptors which increase ventilation if the $P_{CO_2}$ increases. Indeed, often the arterial $P_{CO_2}$ is lower than normal because of the additional hypoxemic stimulus to ventilation.

*Ventilation–Perfusion Inequality*
In this condition, ventilation and blood flow are mismatched in various regions of the lung, with the result that all gas transfer becomes inefficient. This mechanism of hypoxemia is extremely common; it is responsible for most, if not all, of the hypoxemia of COPD, interstitial lung disease, and vascular disorders such as pulmonary embolism. It is often identified by excluding the other three causes of hypoxemia: hypoventilation, diffusion impairment, and shunt.

All lungs have some ventilation–perfusion inequality. In the normal upright lung, this takes the form of a regional pattern, with the ventilation–perfusion ratio decreasing from apex to base. But if pulmonary disease occurs and progresses, we see a disorganization of this pattern until eventually the normal relationships between ventilation and blood flow are destroyed at the alveolar level. (For a discussion of the physiology of how ventilation–perfusion inequality causes hypoxemia, see the companion volume, *Respiratory Physiology: The Essentials*, 9th ed., pp. 66–76.)

Several factors can exaggerate the hypoxemia of ventilation–perfusion inequality. One is concomitant hypoventilation, which may occur, for example, if a patient with severe COPD is overly sedated. Another factor that is frequently overlooked is a reduction in cardiac output. This causes a fall of $P_{O_2}$ in mixed venous blood, which results in a fall of arterial $P_{O_2}$ for the same degree of ventilation–perfusion inequality. This situation may be seen in patients who develop a myocardial infarct with mild pulmonary edema.

How can we assess the severity of ventilation–perfusion inequality from the arterial blood gases? First, the *arterial* $P_{O_2}$ is a useful guide. A patient with an arterial $P_{O_2}$ of 40 mm Hg is likely to have more ventilation–perfusion inequality than a patient with an arterial $P_{O_2}$ of 70 mm Hg. However, we can be misled. For example, suppose that the first patient had reduced the ventilation, with the result that the alveolar $P_{O_2}$ had fallen by 30 mm Hg, thus pulling down the arterial $P_{O_2}$. Under these conditions, the arterial $P_{O_2}$ by itself would be deceptive. For this reason, we often calculate the *alveolar–arterial difference* for $P_{O_2}$.

What value should we use for alveolar $P_{O_2}$? Figure 2-7 reminds us that in a lung with ventilation–perfusion ($\dot{V}_A/\dot{Q}$) inequality, there may be a wide spectrum of values for alveolar $P_{O_2}$ ranging from inspired gas to mixed venous blood. A solution is to calculate an "ideal alveolar $P_{O_2}$." This is the value that the lung *would* have if there were no ventilation–perfusion inequality and if the respiratory exchange ratio remained the same. It is found from the *alveolar gas equation*:

$$P_{A_{O_2}} = P_{I_{O_2}} - \frac{P_{A_{CO_2}}}{R} + F, \qquad \text{(Eq. 2.4)}$$

using the respiratory exchange ratio R of the whole lung, and assuming that arterial and alveolar $P_{CO_2}$ are the same (usually they nearly are). Thus, the alveolar–arterial difference for $P_{O_2}$ makes an allowance for the effect of underventilation or overventilation on the arterial

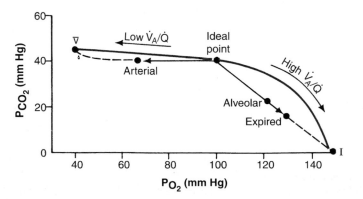

**Figure 2-7. $O_2$–$CO_2$ Diagram Showing the Mixed Venous ($\bar{v}$), Inspired (I), Arterial, Ideal, Alveolar, and Expired Points.** The curved line indicates the $P_{O_2}$ and $P_{CO_2}$ of all lung units having different ventilation–perfusion ($\dot{V}_A/\dot{Q}$) ratios. (For additional information on this difficult topic, see *Respiratory Physiology: The Essentials*, 9th ed., pp. 169–171.)

$P_{O_2}$ and is a purer measure of ventilation–perfusion inequality. Other indices include the physiologic dead space and physiologic shunt. (See *Respiratory Physiology: The Essentials*, 9th ed., pp. 169–171 for further details.)

It is possible to obtain more information about the distribution of ventilation–perfusion ratios in the lung with a technique based on the elimination of injected foreign gases in solution. The details will not be given here, but it is thus possible to derive a virtually continuous distribution of ventilation–perfusion ratios that is consistent with the measured pattern of the elimination of the six gases. Figure 2-8 shows a typical pattern found in young normal volunteers. It can be seen that almost all the ventilation and blood flow go to lung units with ventilation–perfusion ratios near the normal value of 1. As we shall see in Chapter 4, this pattern is greatly disturbed by lung disease.

### Mixed Causes of Hypoxemia

These frequently occur. For example, a patient who is being mechanically ventilated because of acute respiratory failure after an automobile accident may have a large shunt through the unventilated lung in addition to severe ventilation–perfusion inequality (see Figure 8-3). Again, a patient with interstitial lung disease may have some diffusion impairment, but this is certainly accompanied by ventilation–perfusion inequality and possibly by shunt as well (see Figures 5-5 and 5-6). In our present state of knowledge, it is often impossible to define accurately the mechanism of hypoxemia, especially in the serverely ill patient.

### Oxygen Delivery to Tissues

Although the $P_{O_2}$ of arterial blood is of great importance, other factors enter into the delivery of oxygen to the tissues. For example, a reduced arterial $P_{O_2}$ is clearly more detrimental in a patient with a hemoglobin of 5 g/100 ml than it is in a patient with a normal $O_2$ capacity.

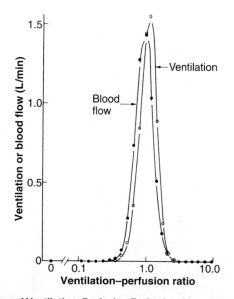

**Figure 2-8. Distribution of Ventilation–Perfusion Ratios in a Young Normal Subject as Obtained by the Multiple Inert Gas Elimination Technique.** Note that most of the ventilation and blood flow go to lung units with ventilation–perfusion ratios near 1. (From Wagner PD, Laravuso RB, Uhl RR, West JB. Continuous distributions of ventilation–perfusion ratios in normal subjects breathing air and 100% $O_2$. *J Clin Invest* 1974;54:54–68.)

The delivery of oxygen to the tissues depends on the oxygen concentration of the blood, the cardiac output, and the distribution of blood flow to the periphery. These factors are discussed further in Chapter 9.

# Arterial $P_{CO_2}$

## Measurement

A $P_{CO_2}$ electrode is essentially a glass pH electrode. This is surrounded by a bicarbonate buffer, which is separated from the blood by a thin membrane through which $CO_2$ diffuses. The $CO_2$ alters the pH of the buffer, and this is measured by the electrode, which reads out the $P_{CO_2}$ directly.

## Normal Values

The normal arterial $P_{CO_2}$ is 37 to 43 mm Hg and is almost unaffected by age. It tends to fall slightly during heavy exercise and to rise slightly during sleep. Sometimes a blood sample obtained by arterial puncture shows a value in the mid-30s. This can be attributed to the acute hyperventilation caused by the procedure and can be recognized by the correspondingly increased pH.

## Causes of Increased Arterial $P_{CO_2}$

There are two major causes of $CO_2$ retention: hypoventilation and ventilation–perfusion inequality.

### Hypoventilation
This was dealt with in some detail earlier in the chapter, where we saw that hypoventilation must cause hypoxemia and $CO_2$ retention, the latter being more important (Figure 2-3). The *alveolar ventilation equation*

$$P_{A_{CO_2}} = \frac{\dot{V}_{CO_2}}{\dot{V}_A} \cdot K, \qquad \text{(Eq. 2.5)}$$

emphasizes the inverse relationship between the ventilation and the alveolar $P_{CO_2}$. In normal lungs, the arterial $P_{CO_2}$ closely follows the alveolar value. Whereas the hypoxemia of hypoventilation can be relieved easily by increasing the inspired $P_{O_2}$, the $CO_2$ retention can only be treated by increasing the ventilation. This may require mechanical assistance as described in Chapter 10.

### Ventilation–Perfusion Inequality
Although this condition was considered earlier, its relationship to $CO_2$ retention warrants a further brief discussion because of frequent confusion in this area. At one time, it was argued that ventilation–perfusion inequality does not interfere with $CO_2$ elimination because the overventilated regions make up for the underventilated areas. This is a fallacy, and it is important to realize that ventilation–perfusion inequality reduces the efficiency of transfer of all gases, including, for example, the anesthetic gases.

Why then do we frequently see patients with chronic pulmonary disease and undoubted ventilation–perfusion inequality who have a normal arterial $P_{CO_2}$ Figure 2-9 explains this. The normal relationships between ventilation and blood flow (A) are disturbed by disease, and hypoxemia and $CO_2$ retention develop (B). However, the chemoreceptors respond to the increased arterial $P_{CO_2}$ and raise the ventilation to the alveoli. The result is that the arterial $P_{CO_2}$ is returned to its normal level (C). However, although the arterial $P_{O_2}$

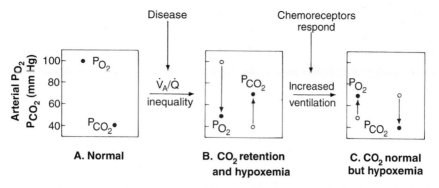

**Figure 2-9. Arterial P$_{O_2}$ and P$_{CO_2}$ in Different Stages of Ventilation–Perfusion Inequality.** Initially there must be both a fall in P$_{O_2}$ and a rise in P$_{CO_2}$. However, when the ventilation to the alveoli is increased, the P$_{CO_2}$ returns to normal but the P$_{O_2}$ remains abnormally low.

is somewhat raised by the increased ventilation, it does not return all the way to normal. This can be explained by the shape of the O$_2$ dissociation curve and, in particular, the strongly depressive action on the arterial P$_{O_2}$ of lung units with low ventilation–perfusion ratios. Whereas units with high ventilation–perfusion ratios are effective at eliminating CO$_2$, they have little advantage over normal units in taking up O$_2$. The end result is that the arterial P$_{CO_2}$ is effectively lowered to the normal value, but there is relatively little rise in arterial P$_{O_2}$.

Some patients do not make the transition from stage B to stage C or, having made it, revert to stage B and develop CO$_2$ retention. What is the reason for this? Generally, these patients have a high work of breathing, often because of a gross increase in airway resistance. Apparently they elect to raise their P$_{CO_2}$ rather than to expend the extra energy to increase ventilation. It is of interest that if normal subjects are made to breathe through a narrow tube, thus increasing their work of breathing, their alveolar P$_{CO_2}$ often rises.

We do not fully understand why some patients with ventilation–perfusion inequality increase their ventilation and some do not. As we shall see in Chapter 5, many patients with emphysema hold their P$_{CO_2}$ at the normal level even when their disease is far advanced. Patients with asthma generally do the same. This can involve a large increase in ventilation to their alveoli. However, other patients, for example, those with severe chronic bronchitis, typically allow their P$_{CO_2}$ to rise much earlier in the course of the disease. It is possible that there is some difference in the central neurogenic control of ventilation in these two groups of patients.

# Arterial pH

## Measurement

Arterial pH is usually measured with a glass electrode concurrently with the arterial P$_{O_2}$ and P$_{CO_2}$. It is related to the P$_{CO_2}$ and bicarbonate concentration through the Henderson-Hasselbalch equation:

$$pH = pK + \log\frac{\left(HCO_3^-\right)}{0.03\, P_{CO_2}} \qquad \text{(Eq. 2.6)}$$

where pK = 6.1, (HCO$_3^-$) is the plasma bicarbonate concentration in millimoles per liter, and the P$_{CO_2}$ is in mm Hg.

## Acidosis

Acidosis is a decrease in arterial pH or a process that tends to do this. Sometimes the term *acidemia* is used to refer to the actual fall in pH in the blood. Acidosis can be caused by respiratory or metabolic abnormalities or by both.

### Respiratory Acidosis

This is caused by $CO_2$ retention, which increases the denominator in the Henderson-Hasselbalch equation and so depresses the pH. Both mechanisms of $CO_2$ retention (hypoventilation and ventilation–perfusion ratio inequality) can cause respiratory acidosis.

It is important to distinguish between acute and chronic $CO_2$ retention. A patient with hypoventilation after an overdose of barbiturate is likely to develop acute respiratory acidosis. There is little change in the bicarbonate concentration (the numerator in the Henderson-Hasselbalch equation), and the pH therefore falls rapidly as the $P_{CO_2}$ rises. Typically, a doubling of the $P_{CO_2}$ from 40 to 80 mm Hg in such a patient reduces the pH from 7.4 to approximately 7.2.

By contrast, a patient who develops chronic $CO_2$ retention over a period of many weeks as a result of increasing ventilation–perfusion inequality caused by chronic pulmonary disease typically has a smaller fall in pH. This is because the kidneys retain bicarbonate in response to the increased $P_{CO_2}$ in the renal tubular cells, thus increasing the numerator in the Henderson-Hasselbalch equation (partially compensated respiratory acidosis).

These relationships are shown diagrammatically in Figure 2-10. Contrast the steep slope of the line for acute $CO_2$ retention (A) with the shallow slope of the line for chronic hypercapnia (B). Note also that a patient with acute hypoventilation whose $P_{CO_2}$ is maintained over 2 or 3 days moves toward the chronic line as the kidney conserves bicarbonate (point *A* to point *C*). Conversely, a patient with COPD with long-standing $CO_2$ retention who develops an acute chest infection with worsening of ventilation–perfusion relationships

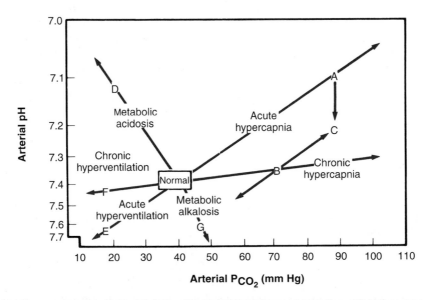

**Figure 2-10. Arterial pH–$P_{CO_2}$ Relationships in Various Types of Acid–Base Disturbances.** (Modified from Flenley DC. Another nonlogarithmic acid–base diagram? *Lancet* 1971;1:961–965.)

may move rapidly from point $B$ to point $C$, that is, parallel to line $A$. However, if he is then mechanically ventilated, he may move back to point $B$, or even beyond.

*Metabolic Acidosis*
This is caused by a primary fall in the numerator ($HCO_3^-$) of the Henderson-Hasselbalch equation, an example being diabetic ketoacidosis. Uncompensated metabolic acidosis would be indicated by a vertical upward movement on Figure 2-10, but in practice the fall in arterial pH stimulates the peripheral chemoreceptors, increasing the ventilation and lowering the $P_{CO_2}$. As a result, the pH and $P_{CO_2}$ move along line $D$.

Lactic acidosis is another form of metabolic acidosis, and this may complicate severe acute respiratory or cardiac failure as a consequence of tissue hypoxia. If such a patient is mechanically ventilated, the pH remains below 7.4 when the $P_{CO_2}$ is returned to normal.

## Alkalosis

Alkalosis (or alkalemia) results from an increase in arterial pH.

*Respiratory Alkalosis*
This is seen in acute hyperventilation where the pH rises, as shown by line $E$ in Figure 2-10. If the hyperventilation is maintained, for example, at high altitude, compensated respiratory alkalosis is seen, with a return of the pH toward normal as the kidney excretes bicarbonate, a movement from point $E$ to point $F$ in Figure 2-10.

*Metabolic Alkalosis*
This is seen in disorders such as severe prolonged vomiting when the plasma bicarbonate concentration rises, as shown by $G$ in Figure 2-10. Usually there is no respiratory compensation but sometimes the $P_{CO_2}$ rises slightly. Metabolic alkalosis also occurs when a patient with long-standing lung disease and compensated respiratory acidosis is ventilated too vigorously, thus bringing the $P_{CO_2}$ rapidly to nearly 40 mm Hg (line $B$ to $G$).

### Four Types of Acid–Base Disturbance

$$pH = pK + \log\frac{HCO_3^-}{0.03\,P_{CO_2}}$$

|  | Primary | Compensation |
|---|---|---|
| **Acidosis** | | |
| Respiratory | $P_{CO_2}$ ↑ | $HCO_3^-$ ↑ |
| Metabolic | $HCO_3^-$ ↓ | $P_{CO_2}$ ↓ |
| **Alkalosis** | | |
| Respiratory | $P_{CO_2}$ ↓ | $HCO_3^-$ ↓ |
| Metabolic | $HCO_3^-$ ↑ | often none |

# Diffusing Capacity

So far, this chapter on gas exchange has been devoted to arterial blood gases and their significance. However, this is a convenient place to discuss another common test of gas exchange—the diffusing capacity of the lung for carbon monoxide.

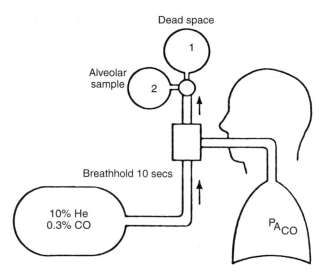

**Figure 2-11. Measurement of the Diffusing Capacity for Carbon Monoxide by the Single-Breath Method.** The subject takes a single breath of 0.3% CO with 10% helium, holds his or her breath for 10 seconds, and then exhales. The first 750 ml is discarded, then an alveolar sample is collected and analyzed.

## Measurement of Diffusing Capacity

The most popular method of measuring the diffusing capacity ($D_{CO}$) is the single-breath method (Figure 2-11). The patient takes a vital capacity breath of 0.3% CO and 10% helium, holds his breath for 10 seconds, and then exhales. The first 750 ml of gas is discarded because of dead space contamination, and the next liter is collected and analyzed. The helium indicates the dilution of the inspired gas with alveolar gas and thus gives the initial alveolar $P_{CO}$. On the assumption that the CO is lost from alveolar gas in proportion to the $P_{CO}$ during breath-holding, the diffusing capacity is calculated as the volume of CO taken up per minute per mm Hg alveolar $P_{CO}$.

## Causes of Reduced Diffusing Capacity

Carbon monoxide is used to measure diffusing capacity because when it is inhaled in low concentrations, the partial pressure in the pulmonary capillary blood remains extremely low in relation to the alveolar value. As a result, CO is taken up by the blood all along the capillary (contrast the time course of $O_2$ shown in Figure 2-4). Thus, the uptake of CO is determined by the *diffusion properties* of the blood–gas barrier and the *rate of combination* of CO with blood.

The diffusion properties of the alveolar membrane depend on its thickness and area. Thus, the diffusing capacity is reduced by diseases in which the thickness is increased, including diffuse interstitial fibrosis, sarcoidosis, and asbestosis (Figure 2-5). It is also reduced when the surface area of the blood–gas barrier is reduced, for example, by pneumonectomy. The fall in diffusing capacity that occurs in emphysema is partly caused by the loss of alveolar walls and capillaries (however, see below).

The rate of combination of CO with blood is reduced when the number of red cells in the capillaries is reduced. This occurs in anemia and in diseases that reduce the capillary blood volume, such as pulmonary embolism. It is possible to separate the membrane and blood component of the diffusing capacity by making the measurement at a high and normal alveolar $P_{O_2}$ (see *Respiratory Physiology: The Essentials*, 9th ed., pp. 33–35).

## Interpretation of Diffusing Capacity

In many patients in whom the measured diffusing capacity is low, the interpretation is uncertain. The reason is the unevenness of ventilation, blood flow, and diffusion properties throughout the diseased lung. We know that such lungs tend to empty unevenly (Figure 1-11), so that the liter of expired gas that is analyzed for CO (Figure 2-11) is probably not representative of the whole lung.

For this reason, the diffusing capacity is sometimes referred to as the *transfer factor* (especially in Europe) to emphasize that it is more a measure of the lung's overall ability to transfer gas into the blood than a specific test of diffusion characteristics. In spite of this uncertainty of interpretation, the test has a definite place in the pulmonary function laboratory and is frequently useful in assessing the severity and type of lung disease.

### Causes of Reduced Diffusing Capacity for Carbon Monoxide

*Blood–gas barrier*
  Thickened in interstitial lung disease
  Area is reduced in emphysema, pneumonectomy
*Capillary blood*
  Volume reduced in pulmonary embolism
  Concentration of red cells reduced in anemia

## KEY CONCEPTS

1. The measurement of arterial blood gases ($P_{O_2}$, $P_{CO_2}$, pH) is relatively simple with modern equipment and is essential in the treatment of patients with respiratory failure.

2. The four causes of hypoxemia are hypoventilation, diffusion impairment, shunt, and ventilation–perfusion inequality. The last is by far the commonest cause.

3. Ventilation–perfusion inequality interferes with the exchange of all gases by the lung including $O_2$ and $CO_2$. All patients with this condition have a reduced arterial $P_{O_2}$, but the $P_{CO_2}$ may be normal if the amount of inspired gas to the alveoli is increased.

4. Acid–base abnormalities include respiratory or metabolic acidosis and respiratory or metabolic alkalosis. These cause characteristic changes in pH, $P_{CO_2}$, and plasma bicarbonate.

5. The diffusing capacity for carbon monoxide is a useful test of gas transfer by the lung.

## QUESTIONS

1. In peripheral capillaries, more oxygen can be unloaded from the blood to the tissues at a given $P_{O_2}$ when:
   A. Blood temperature is reduced.
   B. $P_{CO_2}$ is reduced.
   C. Blood pH is raised.
   D. Concentration of 2,3-DPG in the red cell is raised.
   E. Hydrogen ion concentration is reduced.

2. A young man with normal lungs takes an overdose of barbiturate, which causes him to hypoventilate. Which of the following will probably reach the value of 50 first (assume usual units)?

A. Arterial $P_{O_2}$.
B. Arterial oxygen saturation.
C. Arterial $P_{CO_2}$.
D. Plasma bicarbonate concentration.
E. Base excess.

3. A previously well patient takes an overdose of a narcotic drug and is brought to the emergency room within an hour. The arterial $P_{CO_2}$ is found to be 80 mm Hg. What is the most likely value for the arterial pH?

A. 6.8
B. 7.0
C. 7.2
D. 7.4
E. 7.6

4. A patient with chronic pulmonary disease undergoes emergency surgery. Postoperatively, the arterial $P_{O_2}$, $P_{CO_2}$, and pH are 50 mm Hg, 50 mm Hg, and 7.20, respectively. How would the acid–base status be best described?

A. Mixed respiratory and metabolic acidosis.
B. Uncompensated respiratory acidosis.
C. Fully compensated respiratory acidosis.
D. Uncompensated metabolic acidosis.
E. Fully compensated metabolic acidosis.

5. Which of the following mechanisms of hypoxemia will prevent the arterial $P_{O_2}$ reaching the expected level if the subject is given 100% oxygen to breathe?

A. Hypoventilation.
B. Diffusion impairment.
C. Ventilation–perfusion inequality.
D. Shunt.
E. Residence at high altitude.

6. Concerning obstructive sleep apnea:

A. The condition is rare.
B. All the patients are obese.
C. Treatment by CPAP is often effective.
D. Treatment by CPAP tends to cause systemic hypertension.
E. Snoring is uncommon.

7. Concerning the diffusing capacity of the lung:

A. It is increased in pulmonary fibrosis.
B. Breathing oxygen reduces the measured diffusing capacity for carbon monoxide compared with air breathing.
C. It is increased by pneumonectomy.
D. Diffusion limitation of oxygen transfer during exercise is more likely to occur at sea level than at high altitude.
E. It is best measured with carbon monoxide because this gas diffuses slowly across the blood–gas barrier.

**8.** In a normal person, doubling the diffusing capacity would be expected to:

A. Increase arterial $P_{O_2}$ during moderate exercise.
B. Increase the uptake of halothane given during anesthesia.
C. Decrease arterial $P_{CO_2}$ during resting breathing.
D. Increase resting oxygen uptake when the subject breathes air.
E. Increase maximal oxygen uptake at extreme altitude.

**9.** The laboratory provides the following report on a patient's arterial blood: pH, 7.25; $P_{CO_2}$, 32 mm Hg; and $HCO_3^-$ concentration, 25 mmol·liter$^{-1}$. You conclude that there is:

A. Respiratory alkalosis with metabolic compensation.
B. Acute respiratory acidosis.
C. Metabolic acidosis with respiratory compensation.
D. Metabolic alkalosis with respiratory compensation.
E. A laboratory error.

**10.** An arterial blood sample is taken from a patient with acute shortness of breath breathing air at sea level. Assume the respiratory exchange ratio is 0.8. $P_{O_2} = 70$ torr, $P_{CO_2} = 32$ torr, pH = 7.30. These data indicate:

A. A primary respiratory alkalosis with metabolic compensation.
B. A normal alveolar–arterial $P_{O_2}$ difference.
C. An arterial $O_2$ saturation of less than 70%.
D. The sample was mistakenly drawn from a vein.
E. A partially compensated metabolic acidosis.

# Other Tests

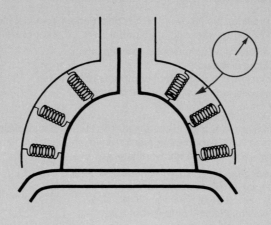

In Chapters 1 and 2, we concentrated on two simple but informative tests of pulmonary function: forced expiration and arterial blood gases. In this chapter, we briefly consider some other ways of measuring lung function. Of the large number of possible tests that have been introduced from time to time, we address only the most useful here and emphasize the principles rather than the details of their use.

## ▶ Static Lung Volumes

### Measurement

The measurement of the vital capacity with a simple spirometer was described in Chapter 1 (Figure 1-1). This equipment can also be used to obtain the tidal volume, vital capacity, and expiratory reserve volume (functional residual capacity minus the residual volume). However, the residual volume, functional residual capacity, and total lung capacity require additional measurements.

The functional residual capacity (FRC) can be measured with a body plethysmograph, which is essentially a large airtight box in which the patient sits. (See *Respiratory Physiology: The Essentials*, 9th ed., p. 16.) The mouthpiece is obstructed and the patient is instructed to make a rapid inspiratory effort. As he expands the gas volume in the lungs, the air in the plethysmograph is compressed slightly and its pressure rises. By applying Boyle's law, the lung volume can be obtained. Another method is to use the helium dilution technique, in which a spirometer of known volume and helium concentration is connected to the patient in a closed circuit. From the degree of dilution of the helium, the unknown lung volume can be calculated. The residual volume can be derived from the FRC by subtracting the expiratory reserve volume.

### Interpretation

The FRC and RV are typically increased in diseases in which there is an increased airway resistance, for example, emphysema, chronic bronchitis, and asthma. Indeed, at one time, an elevated RV was regarded as an essential feature of emphysema. The RV is raised in these conditions because airway closure occurs at an abnormally high lung volume.

A reduced FRC and RV are often seen in patients with reduced lung compliance, for example, in diffuse interstitial fibrosis. In this case, the lung is stiff and tends to recoil to a smaller resting volume.

If the FRC is measured by both the plethysmographic and gas dilution methods, a comparison of the two results is often informative. The plethysmographic method measures all the gas in the lung. However, the dilution technique "sees" only those regions of lung that communicate with the mouth. Therefore, regions behind closed airways (e.g., some cysts) result in a higher value for the plethysmographic than for the dilution procedure. The same disparity is often seen in patients with chronic obstructive pulmonary disease, probably because some areas are so poorly ventilated that they do not equilibrate in the time allowed.

## ▶ Lung Elasticity

### Measurement

The pressure-volume curve of the lung requires knowledge of the pressures both in the airways and around the lung (see *Respiratory Physiology: The Essentials*, 9th ed., p. 102). A good estimate of the latter can be obtained from the esophageal pressure. A small balloon at the end of a catheter is passed down through the nose or mouth, and the difference between the mouth and esophageal pressures is recorded as the patient exhales in steps of 1 liter from TLC to RV. The resulting pressure-volume curve is not linear (Figure 3-1), so that a single value for its slope (compliance) can be misleading. However, the compliance is sometimes reported for the liter above FRC measured on the descending limb of the pressure-volume curve.

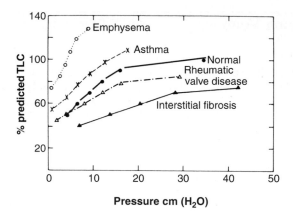

**Figure 3-1. Pressure-Volume Curves of the Lung.** Note that the curves for emphysema and asthma (during an attack) are shifted upward and to the left, whereas those for rheumatic valve disease and interstitial fibrosis are flattened. (From Bates DV, Macklem PT, Christie RV. *Respiratory Function in Disease.* 2nd ed. Philadelphia, PA: WB Saunders, 1971.)

The pressure-volume curve is often reported using the percentage of predicted TLC on the vertical axis rather than using the actual lung volume in liters (Figure 3-1). This procedure helps to allow for differences in body size and reduces the variability of the results.

## Interpretation

Elastic recoil is *reduced* in patients with emphysema. Figure 3-1 shows that the pressure-volume curve is displaced to the left and has a steeper slope in this condition as a result of the destruction of the alveolar walls (see also Figures 4-2, 4-3, and 4-5) and the consequent disorganization of elastic tissue. The change in compliance is not reversible. The pressure-volume curve is also typically shifted to the left in patients who are having an asthma attack, but the change is reversible in some patients. The reasons for this shift are unclear. Increasing age also tends to reduce elastic recoil.

| Some Conditions Affecting Lung Elasticity | |
|---|---|
| Elastic recoil is *reduced* in | emphysema |
| | some patients with asthma |
| Elastic recoil is *increased* by | interstitial fibrosis |
| | interstitial edema |

Elastic recoil is *increased* in interstitial fibrosis, which results in the deposition of fibrous tissue in the alveolar walls (see Figures 2-5 and 5-3), thus reducing the lung's distensibility. Elastic recoil also tends to increase in patients with rheumatic heart disease who have a raised pulmonary capillary pressure and some interstitial edema. However, note that measurements of the pressure-volume curve show considerable variability, and the neat results shown in Figure 3-1 are based on mean values from many patients.

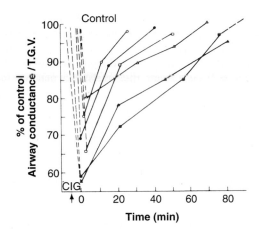

**Figure 3-2. Effect of Cigarette Smoking on Airway Conductance as Measured in the Body Plethysmograph.** The ordinate shows conductance related to thoracic gas volume. (From Nadel JA, Comroe Jr, JH. Acute effects of inhalation of cigarette smoke on airway conductance. *J Appl Physiol* 1961;16:713–716.)

## ▶ Airway Resistance

### Measurement

Airway resistance is measured as the pressure difference between the alveoli and the mouth divided by the flow rate. Alveolar pressure can only be measured indirectly: one way to do this is with a body plethysmograph. (See *Respiratory Physiology: The Essentials*, 9th ed., p. 174.) The subject sits in an airtight box and pants through a flow meter. The alveolar pressure can be deduced from the pressure changes in the plethysmograph because when the alveolar gas is compressed, the plethysmograph gas volume increases slightly, causing a fall in pressure. This method has the advantage that lung volume can be measured easily almost simultaneously. Figure 3-2 shows the effect of cigarette smoking on airway resistance, here expressed as its reciprocal, *conductance*.

### Interpretation

Airway resistance is reduced by an increase in lung volume because the expanding parenchyma exerts traction on the airway walls. Thus, any measurement of airway resistance must be related to the lung volume. Note that the small peripheral airways normally contribute little to overall resistance because there are so many arranged in parallel. For this reason, special tests have been devised to try to detect early changes in small airways. These changes include the flow rate during the latter part of the flow-volume curve (see Figure 1-8) and closing volume (see Figure 1-10).

| Some Conditions Affecting Airway Resistance | |
|---|---|
| Resistance is *increased* by | chronic bronchitis |
| | asthma |
| | emphysema |
| | inhaled irritants (e.g., cigarette smoke) |
| Resistance is *decreased* by | increased lung volume |

Airway resistance is *increased* in chronic bronchitis and emphysema. In chronic bronchitis, the lumen of a typical airway contains excessive secretions and the wall is thickened by mucous gland hyperplasia and edema (see Figure 4-6). In emphysema, many of the airways lose the radical traction of the tissue surrounding them because of destruction of the alveolar walls (see Figures 4-1 and 4-2). As a result, their resistance may not increase much during quiet breathing (it may be nearly normal), but with any exertion, dynamic compression (see Figure 1-6) quickly occurs on expiration, and resistance rises strikingly. Such patients often show a reasonably high flow rate early in expiration, but this abruptly drops to low values as flow limitation occurs (see the flow-volume curve in Figure 1-8). Recall that the driving pressure under these conditions is the static recoil pressure of the lung (see Figure 1-6), which is reduced in emphysema (Figure 3-1).

Airway resistance is also increased in patients with bronchial asthma. Here the factors include contraction of bronchial smooth muscle with resultant bronchoconstriction, mucous plugs occluding many of the airways, and edema of their walls (see Figure 4-13). The resistance may be high during attacks, especially in relation to lung volume, which is frequently greatly increased. The resistance is reduced by bronchodilator drugs such as β2-agonists. Even during periods of remission when the patient is asymptomatic, airway resistance is often raised.

Tracheal obstruction increases airway resistance. This may be caused by compression from outside, for example, an enlarged thyroid, or by intrinsic narrowing caused by scarring or a tumor (fixed obstruction). An important feature is that the obstruction is usually apparent during *inspiration* and it can be detected on an inspiratory flow-volume curve (see Figure 1-9). In addition, an audible stridor may be present.

## ▶ Control of Ventilation

## Measurement

The ventilatory response to carbon dioxide can be measured with a rebreathing technique. A small bag is filled with a mixture of 6-7% $CO_2$ in oxygen, and the patient rebreathes from this over a period of several minutes. The bag $P_{CO_2}$ increases at the rate of 4 to 6 mm Hg/min because of the $CO_2$ being produced from the tissues, and thus the change in ventilation per mm Hg increase in $P_{CO_2}$ can be determined.

The ventilatory response to hypoxia can be measured in a similar way. In this instance, the bag is filled with 24% $O_2$, 7% $CO_2$, and the balance with $N_2$. During rebreathing, the $P_{CO_2}$ is monitored and held constant by means of a variable bypass and $CO_2$ absorber. As the oxygen is taken up, the increase in ventilation is related to the $P_{O_2}$ in the bag and lungs.

Both these techniques give information about the overall ventilatory response to $CO_2$ or hypoxia, but they do not differentiate between patients who *will not* breathe because of central nervous system or neuromuscular inadequacy and those who *cannot* breathe because of mechanical abnormalities of the chest. To make this distinction between those who "won't" and those who "can't" breathe, the mechanical work done during inspiration can be measured. To accomplish this, the esophageal pressure is recorded with tidal volume, and the area of the pressure-volume loop is obtained. (See *Respiratory Physiology: The Essentials*, 9th ed., p. 125). Inspiratory work recorded in this way is one useful measure of the neural output of the respiratory center.

## Interpretation

The ventilatory response to $CO_2$ is depressed by sleep, narcotic drugs, and genetic, racial, and personality factors. An important question is why some patients with chronic pulmonary disease develop $CO_2$ retention and others do not. In this context, considerable differences of

$CO_2$ response exist among individuals, and it has been suggested that the course of patients with chronic respiratory disease may be related to this factor. Thus, patients who respond strongly to a rise in $P_{CO_2}$ may be more distressed by dyspnea, whereas those who respond weakly may allow their $P_{CO_2}$ to rise and they succumb to respiratory failure.

The factors that affect the ventilatory response to hypoxia are less clearly understood. However, the response is reduced in many persons who have been hypoxemic since birth, such as those born at high altitude or with cyanotic congenital heart disease. The hypoxic ventilatory response tends to be preserved during sleep. However, some patients develop sleep apnea syndromes, as discussed in Chapter 2.

## ▶ Exercise Tests

### Measurement

The normal lung has enormous reserves of function at rest. For example, the $O_2$ uptake and $CO_2$ output can be increased 10-fold or more when a normal person exercises, and these increases occur without a fall in arterial $P_{O_2}$ or a rise in $P_{CO_2}$. Therefore, to reveal minor dysfunction, the stress of exercise is often useful.

Another reason for exercise testing is to assess disability. Patients vary considerably in their own assessment of the amount of activity they can do, and an objective measurement on a treadmill, stationary bicycle, or a walk along a hallway can be revealing. Occasionally, exercise tests are diagnostic, for example, in exercise-induced asthma and in myocardial ischemia causing angina. Exercise tests can help evaluate the cause of dyspnea.

The variables that are often measured during exercise include work load, total ventilation, respiratory frequency, tidal volume, heart rate, ECG, blood pressure, $O_2$ uptake, $CO_2$ output, arterial $P_{O_2}$, $P_{CO_2}$, and pH. More specialized measurements, such as diffusing capacity, cardiac output, and blood lactate concentration, are sometimes made. Abnormal gas exchange can be characterized by the physiologic dead space and shunt as at rest.

Less formal exercise tests (so-called field exercise tests) can also be informative. One is the 6-minute walk test (6MWT), in which the patient is asked to walk as far as possible along a corridor or other flat terrain for 6 minutes. The result is expressed in meters covered and has the advantage that the test simulates real-life conditions. The results often improve with practice. Another test is the shuttle walk test, in which the patient walks around two cones placed 10 meters apart. The walking speed is controlled by an audiotape that "beeps" and the walking speed is successively increased.

### Interpretation

In most instances, the interpretation of the tests during exercise is similar to that of tests done at rest except that exercise exaggerates the abnormalities. For example, a patient with interstitial lung disease who has a marginally reduced diffusing capacity at rest may show almost no increase on exercise (an abnormal result), with a marked fall in arterial $P_{O_2}$, a relatively small rise in cardiac output, and perhaps striking dyspnea. Figure 3-3B shows the exercise response of a patient with hypersensitivity pneumonitis. Note the rapid increase in ventilation at relatively low work levels and the fall in arterial $P_{O_2}$ and $P_{CO_2}$.

Some investigators take special note of the respiratory exchange ratio (R) as the exercise level is increased, although this requires special equipment for its continuous measurement. When the patient reaches the limit of his or her steady-state aerobic exercise (sometimes called the *anaerobic threshold* or *ventilation threshold*), the R rises more rapidly. This is caused by an increase in the $CO_2$ production secondary to the liberation of lactic acid from the

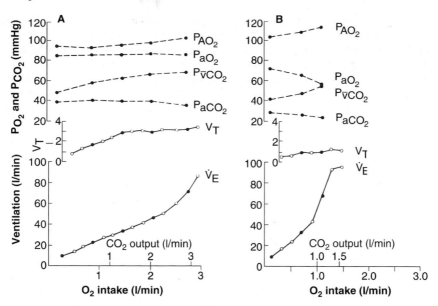

**Figure 3-3. Results Obtained During Exercise Testing. A.** Normal pattern. **B.** Results in a patient with hypersensitivity pneumonitis. Note the restricted work level evidenced by the limited $O_2$ intake, the excessive ventilation for the $O_2$ intake, and the marked fall in arterial $P_{O_2}$. (From Jones NL. Exercise testing in pulmonary evaluation. *N Engl J Med* 1975;293:541–544, 647–650.)

hypoxic muscles. The hydrogen ions react with bicarbonate and lead to an increase in $CO_2$ excretion above that produced by aerobic metabolism. The fall in pH provides an additional stimulus to breathing.

Sometimes it is possible to identify the chief factor limiting exercise in a patient with mixed disease. For example, patients who have both heart and lung disease present a common problem. Exercise testing may reveal that at a patient's maximum work load there is abnormal pulmonary gas exchange with a high physiologic dead space and shunt, suggesting that the patient's lung is the weak link. Alternatively, the cardiac output may respond poorly to exercise, thus suggesting heart disease as the chief culprit. Sometimes, however, the interpretation is not clear-cut.

## ▶ Dyspnea

*Dyspnea* refers to the sensation of difficulty with breathing, and it should be distinguished from simple tachypnea (rapid breathing) or hyperpnea (increased ventilation). Because dyspnea is a subjective phenomenon, it is difficult to measure, and the factors responsible for it are poorly understood. Broadly speaking, dyspnea occurs when the *demand for ventilation* is out of proportion to the patient's *ability to respond* to that demand. As a result, breathing becomes difficult, uncomfortable, or labored.

An *increased demand for ventilation* is often caused by changes in the blood gases and pH level. High ventilations on exercise are common in patients with inefficient pulmonary gas exchange, especially those with large physiologic dead spaces, who tend to develop $CO_2$ retention and acidosis unless they achieve high ventilations. Another important factor is stimulation of intrapulmonary receptors. This factor presumably explains the high exercise ventilations in many patients with interstitial lung disease, possibly as a result of stimulation of the juxtacapillary (J) receptors (Figure 3-3B).

A *reduced ability to respond* to the ventilatory needs is generally caused by abnormal mechanics of the lung or chest wall. Frequently, increased airway resistance is the problem, as in asthma, but other causes include a stiff chest wall, as in kyphoscoliosis.

The assessment of dyspnea is difficult. One way is to ask the patient to indicate his or her perceived feeling of dyspnea on a linear scale from 1 to 10, with 1 being the lowest and 10 the highest. This type of measurement is especially useful before and after an intervention such as treatment with a bronchodilator. Exercise tolerance is often determined from a standard questionnaire that grades breathlessness according to how far the patient can walk on the level or go upstairs without pausing for breath. Occasionally, in an attempt to obtain an index of dyspnea, ventilation is measured at a standard level of exercise and is then related to the patient's maximum voluntary ventilation. However, dyspnea is something that only the patient feels; as such, it cannot be measured objectively.

## ▶ Topographic Differences of Lung Function

### Measurement

The regional distribution of blood flow and ventilation in the lung can be measured with radioactive substances (see *Respiratory Physiology: The Essentials*, 9th ed., pp. 23, 46). One method of detecting areas of absent blood flow is by injecting albumin aggregates labeled with radioactive technetium. An image of the radioactivity is then made with a gamma camera, and "cold" areas containing no activity are readily apparent. A major application of this method in practice is the diagnosis of pulmonary embolism.

The distribution of blood flow can also be obtained from an intravenous injection of radioactive xenon or other gas dissolved in saline. When the gas reaches the pulmonary capillaries, it is evolved into the alveolar gas, and the radiation can be detected by a gamma camera. This method has the advantage of giving blood flow per unit volume of lung.

The distribution of ventilation can be measured in a similar way, except that the gas is inhaled into the alveoli from a spirometer. Either a single inspiration or a wash-in over a series of breaths can be recorded.

### Interpretation

The distribution of blood flow in the upright lung is uneven, being much greater at the base than at the apex (Figure 3-4). The differences are caused by gravity and can be explained by the relationships between the pulmonary arterial, venous, and alveolar pressures. (See *Respiratory Physiology: The Essentials*, 9th ed., p. 47.) Exercise results in a more uniform distribution because of the increase in pulmonary arterial pressure; the same result is found in disease conditions such as pulmonary hypertension and left-to-right cardiac shunts. Localized lung disease, for example, a cyst, or area of fibrosis, frequently decreases regional blood flow.

The distribution of ventilation is also gravity-dependent, and normally the ventilation to the base exceeds that to the apex. The explanation is the distortion that the lung suffers because of gravity and the larger transpulmonary pressure at the apex compared with the base. (See *Respiratory Physiology: The Essentials*, 9th ed., p. 109). Localized lung disease, for example, a bulla, usually reduces the ventilation in that area. In generalized lung diseases—such as asthma, chronic bronchitis, emphysema, and interstitial fibrosis—areas of reduced ventilation and blood flow can frequently be detected.

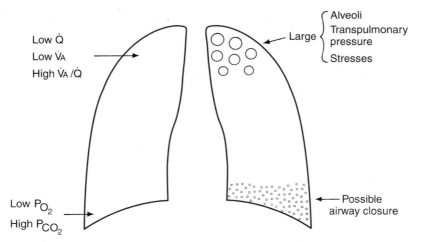

**Figure 3-4. Regional Differences of Structure and Function in the Upright Lung.**

Healthy people show a reversal of the normal pattern of ventilation if they inhale a small amount of radioactive gas from residual volume. The reason is that the airways at the base of the lung are closed under these conditions because intrapleural pressure actually rises above airway pressure. The same pattern may occur at FRC in older subjects because the lower-zone airways close at an abnormally high lung volume. Similar findings may be seen in patients with emphysema, interstitial edema, and obesity. All these conditions exaggerate airway closure at the base of the lung.

Other regional differences of structure and function also occur. The gravity-induced distortion of the upright lung causes the alveoli at the apex to be larger than those at the base. These larger alveoli are also associated with greater mechanical stresses that may play a role in the development of some diseases, such as centriacinar emphysema (see Figure 4-5A) and spontaneous pneumothorax.

## ▶ Value of Pulmonary Function Tests

Because this book is about the function of diseased lungs, it is natural that we should start with pulmonary function tests. However, it is important to recognize that these tests have a limited role in clinical practice. They are rarely useful in making a specific diagnosis; rather, they provide supporting information that is added to that obtained from the clinical history, physical examination, chest imaging, and laboratory tests. Lung function tests are particularly valuable in following the progress of a patient, for example, assessing the efficacy of bronchodilator therapy in a patient with asthma. They are also useful in assessing patients for surgery, determining disability for purposes of workers' compensation, and estimating the prevalence of disease in a community, for example, in a coal mine or an asbestos factory. Lung function tests are occasionally within normal limits despite obvious generalized lung diseases.

As has been emphasized, spirometry gives useful information with simple equipment. Arterial blood gases are more difficult to measure, but the data may be lifesaving for patients with respiratory failure. The value of the other tests depends largely on the clinical problem, and whether they are worth doing is related to the facilities of the pulmonary function laboratory, the expense, and the likelihood that they will give useful information.

## KEY CONCEPTS

1. Lung elastic recoil is reduced in emphysema and some patients with asthma. It is increased in interstitial fibrosis and slightly in interstitial edema.

2. Airway resistance is increased in chronic bronchitis, emphysema, and asthma. It is reduced by increasing lung volume. Tracheal obstruction increases both inspiratory and expiratory resistance.

3. The control of ventilation by increased $P_{CO_2}$ and reduced $P_{O_2}$ varies greatly among people and may affect the clinical pattern of COPD.

4. The lung at rest has enormous reserves of function, and valuable information can therefore often be obtained during exercise that stresses gas exchange.

5. Dyspnea is a common, important symptom in many lung diseases but can be truly assessed only by the patient.

## QUESTIONS

1. The functional residual capacity:
   A. Can be measured with a single spirometer.
   B. Is often larger when measured by helium dilution than with a body plethysmograph.
   C. Is reduced during an attack of asthma.
   D. Is determined by a balance between the elastic recoil of the lung and chest wall.
   E. Falls with increasing age.

2. Airway resistance in a patient with asthma:
   A. Is raised by increasing lung volume.
   B. Is reduced by inhaling $\beta_2$-agonists.
   C. Is increased by destruction of alveolar walls.
   D. Is unaffected by secretions in the airways.
   E. Is increased by loss of bronchial smooth muscle.

3. During an exercise test on a patient with mitral stenosis, it was found that the respiratory exchange ratio of expired gas rapidly rose above 1 at a low level of exercise. A likely reason is:
   A. Abnormally high levels of lactate in the blood.
   B. Abnormally low ventilation.
   C. Abnormally high cardiac output.
   D. Increased lung compliance.
   E. Reduced diffusing capacity of the lung.

4. In the upright human lung, which of the following is greater at the apex than the base?
   A. Blood flow.
   B. Ventilation.
   C. Alveolar $P_{CO_2}$.
   D. Alveolar size.
   E. Capillary blood volume.

5. Which of the following increases *by the largest percentage* at maximal exercise compared with rest?
   A. $P_{CO_2}$ of mixed venous blood.
   B. Alveolar ventilation.
   C. Tidal volume.
   D. Heart rate.
   E. Cardiac output.

# PART TWO

# Function of the Diseased Lung

This part is devoted to the patterns of abnormal function in some common types of lung disease.

# Obstructive Diseases

**4**

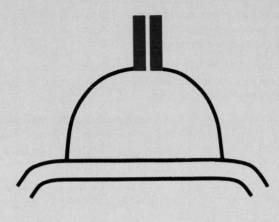

O bstructive diseases of the lung are extremely common. In the United States, they are second only to heart disease as a cause of disability benefits from the Social Security Administration. They are also becoming increasingly important as a cause of mortality. Unfortunately, as we will see, the distinctions among the various types of obstructive disease are blurred, giving rise to difficulties in definition and diagnosis. However, all these diseases are characterized by airway obstruction.

47

## ▶ Airway Obstruction

Increased resistance to airflow can be caused by conditions (1) inside the lumen, (2) in the wall of the airway, and (3) in the peribronchial region (Figure 4-1):

**1.** The lumen may be partially occluded by excessive secretions, such as in chronic bronchitis. Partial obstruction can also occur acutely in pulmonary edema or after aspiration of foreign material and, postoperatively, with retained secretions. Inhaled foreign bodies may cause localized partial or complete obstruction.

**2.** Causes in the wall of the airway include contraction of bronchial smooth muscle, as in asthma; hypertrophy of the mucous glands, as in chronic bronchitis (see Figure 4-6); and inflammation and edema of the wall, as in bronchitis and asthma.

**3.** Outside the airway, destruction of lung parenchyma may cause loss of radial traction and consequent narrowing, as in emphysema. A bronchus may also be compressed locally by an enlarged lymph node or neoplasm. Peribronchial edema can also cause narrowing (see Figure 6-5).

## ▶ Chronic Obstructive Pulmonary Disease

Chronic obstructive pulmonary disease (COPD) is an ill-defined term that is often applied to patients who have emphysema, chronic bronchitis, or a mixture of the two. Many patients who report increasing shortness of breath over several years are found to have a chronic cough, poor exercise tolerance, evidence of airway obstruction, overinflated lungs, and impaired gas exchange. It is often difficult to know to what extent these patients have emphysema or chronic bronchitis, and the term "chronic obstructive pulmonary disease" is a convenient, nondescript label that avoids making an unwarranted diagnosis with inadequate data.

### Emphysema

*Emphysema is characterized by enlargement of the air spaces distal to the terminal bronchiole, with destruction of their walls. Note that this is an anatomic definition; in other words, the diagnosis is presumptive in the living patient.*

### Pathology

A typical histologic appearance is shown in Figure 4-2B. Note that, in contrast to the normal lung section in Figure 4-2A, the emphysematous lung shows loss of alveolar walls with

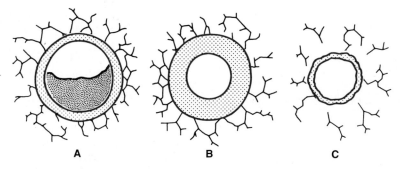

**Figure 4-1. Mechanisms of Airway Obstruction. A.** The lumen is partly blocked, for example, by excessive secretions. **B.** The airway wall is thickened, for example, by edema or hypertrophy of smooth muscle. **C.** The abnormality is outside the airway; in this example, the lung parenchyma is partly destroyed and the airway has narrowed because of the loss of radial traction.

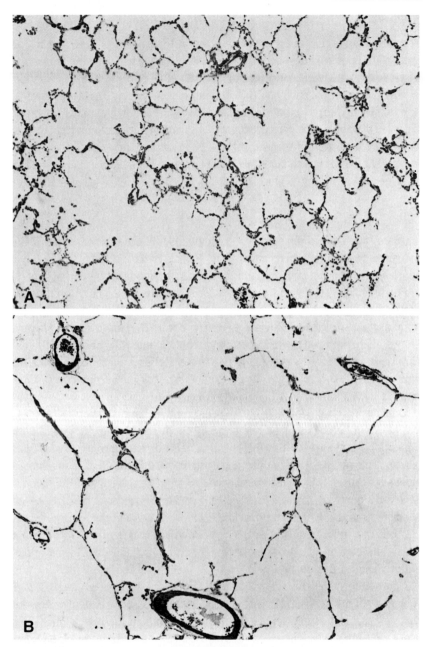

**Figure 4-2. Microscopic Appearance of Emphysematous Lung. A.** Normal lung. **B.** Loss of alveolar walls and consequent enlargement of airspaces (× 90). (From Heard BE. *Pathology of Chronic Bronchitis and Emphysema.* London, UK: Churchill, 1969.)

consequent destruction of parts of the capillary bed. Strands of parenchyma that contain blood vessels can sometimes be seen coursing across large dilated airspaces. The small airways (<2 mm wide) are narrowed, tortuous, and reduced in number. In addition, they have thin, atrophied walls. There is also some loss of larger airways. The structural changes are well seen with the naked eye or hand lens in large slices of lung (Figure 4-3).

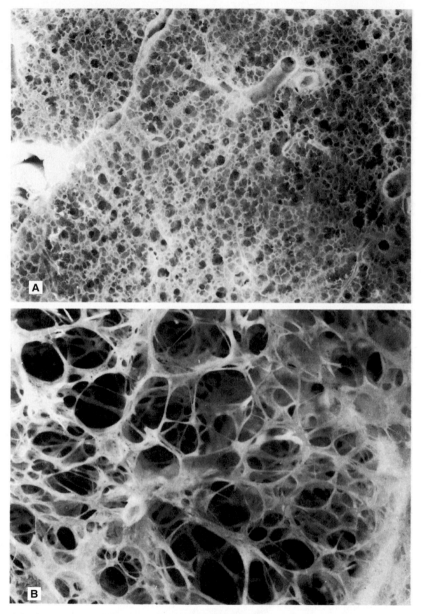

**Figure 4-3. Appearance of Slices of Normal and Emphysematous Lung. A.** Normal. **B.** Panacinar emphysema (barium sulfate impregnation, × 14). (From Heard BE. *Pathology of Chronic Bronchitis and Emphysema.* London, UK: Churchill, 1969.)

## *Types*

Various types of emphysema are recognized. The definition given earlier indicates that the disease affects the parenchyma distal to the terminal bronchiole. This unit is the *acinus*, but it may not be damaged uniformly. In *centriacinar emphysema*, the destruction is limited to the central part of the lobule, and the peripheral alveolar ducts and alveoli may escape unscathed (Figure 4-4).

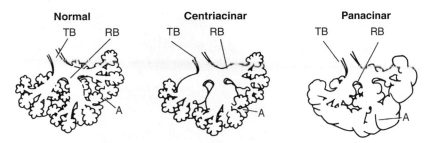

**Figure 4-4. Centriacinar and Panacinar Emphysema.** In centriacinar emphysema, the destruction is confined to the terminal and respiratory bronchioles (TB and RB). In panacinar emphysema, the peripheral alveoli (A) are also involved.

By contrast, *panacinar emphysema* shows distension and destruction of the whole lobule. Occasionally the disease is most marked in the lung adjacent to interlobular septa (paraseptal emphysema). In other patients, large cystic areas or bullae develop (bullous emphysema).

Centriacinar and panacinar emphysema tend to have different topographic distributions. The former is typically most marked in the apex of the upper lobe but spreads down the lung as the disease progresses (Figure 4-5A). The predilection for the apex might reflect the higher mechanical stresses (see Figure 3-4), which predispose to structural failure of the alveolar walls. By contrast, panacinar emphysema has no regional preference or, possibly, is more common in the lower lobes. When emphysema is severe, it is difficult to distinguish the two types, and these may coexist in one lung. The centriacinar form is extremely common, and mild forms apparently cause no dysfunction.

Another form of emphysema is that associated with $\alpha_1$-antitrypsin deficiency. Patients who are homozygous for the Z gene frequently develop severe panacinar emphysema, which usually begins in the lower lobes (Figure 4-5B). The disease may become evident by the age of 40 years and often occurs without cough or smoking history. Therapy by replacement of $\alpha_1$-antitrypsin is now available. Heterozygotes do not seem to be at risk, although this is not certain. Other variants of emphysema include unilateral emphysema (MacLeod's or Swyer-James syndrome), which causes a unilaterally hyperlucent chest radiograph.

## Pathogenesis

This is an active area of research. One current hypothesis is that excessive amounts of the enzyme lysosomal elastase are released from the neutrophils in the lung. This results in the destruction of elastin, an important structural protein of the lung. Neutrophil elastase also cleaves type IV collagen, and this molecule is important in determining the strength of the thin side of the pulmonary capillary and therefore the integrity of the alveolar wall. Animals that have had neutrophil elastase instilled into their airways develop histologic changes that are similar in many ways to emphysema.

Cigarette smoking is an important pathogenic factor and may work by stimulating macrophages to release neutrophil chemoattractants, such as C5a, or by reducing the activity of elastase inhibitors. In addition, many neutrophils are normally marginated (trapped) in the lung, and this process is exaggerated by cigarette smoking, which also activates trapped leucocytes.

This hypothesis puts the etiology on the same footing as that for the emphysema of $\alpha_1$-antitrypsin deficiency, in which the mechanism is the lack of the antiprotease that normally inhibits elastase. One puzzle is why some heavy smokers do not develop the disease. Air pollution may play a role, as may hereditary factors, which are clearly important in $\alpha_1$-antitrypsin deficiency.

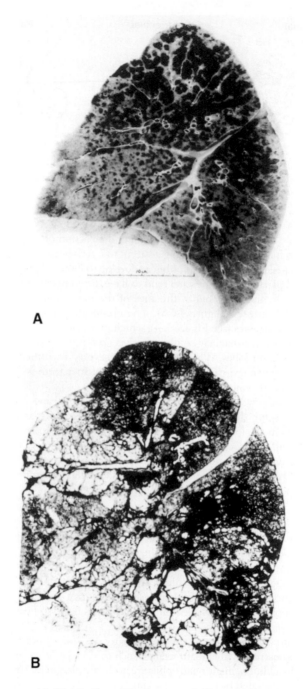

**Figure 4-5. Topographic Distribution of Emphysema. A.** The typical upper zone preference of centriacinar emphysema. **B.** The typical lower zone preference of emphysema caused by $\alpha_1$-antitrypsin deficiency. (From Heard BE. *Pathology of Chronic Bronchitis and Emphysema.* London, UK: Churchill, 1969.)

# Chronic Bronchitis

*This disease is characterized by excessive mucus production in the bronchial tree, sufficient to cause excessive expectoration of sputum. Note that this is a clinical definition (unlike the definition of emphysema). In practice, criteria for excessive expectoration are often laid down, for example, expectoration on most days for at least 3 months in the year for at least 2 successive years.*

## Pathology

The hallmark is hypertrophy of mucous glands in the large bronchi (Figure 4-6) and evidence of chronic inflammatory changes in the small airways. The mucous gland enlargement

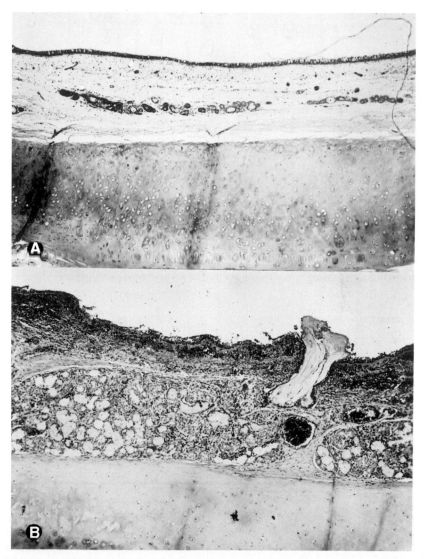

**Figure 4-6. Histologic Changes in Chronic Bronchitis. A.** A normal bronchial wall. **B.** Bronchial wall of a patient with chronic bronchitis. Note the great hypertrophy of the mucous glands, the thickened submucosa, and the cellular infiltration (3 × 60). Compare with the diagram of the bronchial wall in Figure 4-7. (From Thurlbeck WM. *Chronic Airflow Obstruction in Lung Disease.* Philadelphia, PA: WB Saunders, 1976.)

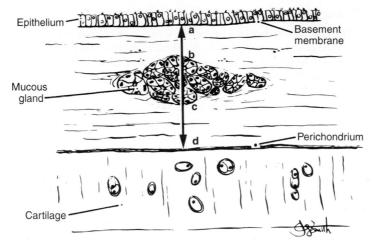

**Figure 4-7. Structure of a Normal Bronchial Wall.** In chronic bronchitis, the thickness of the mucous glands increases and can be expressed as the Reid index given by (b-c)/(a-d). (From Thurlbeck WM. *Chronic Airflow Obstruction in Lung Disease.* Philadelphia, PA: WB Saunders, 1976.)

may be expressed as the gland–wall ratio, which is normally <0.4 but may exceed 0.7 in severe chronic bronchitis. This is known as the "Reid index" (Figure 4-7). Excessive amounts of mucus are found in the airways, and semisolid plugs of mucus may occlude some small bronchi.

In addition, the small airways are narrowed and show inflammatory changes, including cellular infiltration and edema of the walls. Granulation tissue is present, and peribronchial fibrosis may develop. Apparently, bronchial smooth muscle increases. There is evidence that the initial pathologic changes are in the small airways and that these progress to the larger bronchi.

### *Pathogenesis*

Again, cigarette smoking is the chief culprit. Repeated exposure to this inhaled irritant results in chronic inflammation. If you hear a patient give a moist fruity cough, you can safely bet that he is a smoker. Air pollution caused by smog or industrial smoke is another definite factor.

## Clinical Features of Chronic Obstructive Pulmonary Disease

As we have seen, chronic bronchitis is a clinical definition, and the diagnosis in the living patient can therefore be made confidently. However, a definitive diagnosis of emphysema requires histologic confirmation that is usually not available during life, although a combination of history, physical examination, and radiology (especially computed tomography [CT]) can give a high probability of the diagnosis. It follows that the amount of emphysema in a given patient is uncertain. This is why COPD remains a useful term.

Within the spectrum of COPD, two extremes of clinical presentation are recognized: type A and type B. At one time it was thought that these types correlated to some extent with the relative amounts of emphysema and chronic bronchitis, respectively, in the lung, but this view has been challenged. Nevertheless, it is still useful to describe two patterns of clinical presentation because they represent different pathophysiologies. In practice, most patients have features of both.

## Type A

A typical presentation would be a man in his middle 50s who has had increasing shortness of breath for the last 3 or 4 years. Cough may be absent or may produce little white sputum. Physical examination reveals an asthenic build with evidence of recent weight loss. There is no cyanosis. The chest is overexpanded with quiet breath sounds and no adventitious sounds. The radiograph (Figure 4-8B) confirms the overinflation with low diaphragms, narrow mediastinum, and increased retrosternal translucency (between the sternum and the heart on the lateral view). In addition, the radiograph shows attenuation and narrowing of the peripheral pulmonary vessels. Additional information is available from computer tomography (CT). Figure 4-9A shows a normal lung using this digital technique, and the fine resolution can be seen. Figure 4-9B shows an axial section of a lung from a patient with emphysema. Holes scattered throughout the lung can be seen. These patients have been dubbed "pink puffers."

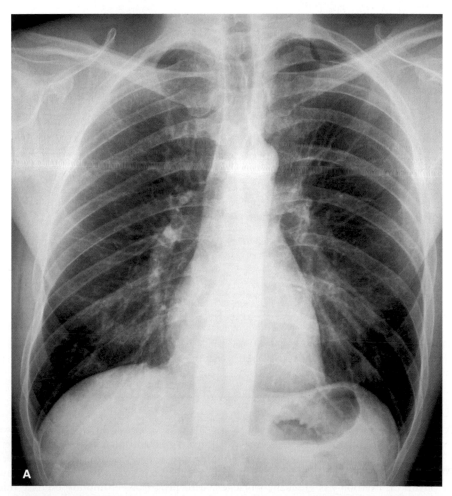

**Figure 4-8.** Radiographic Appearances in the Normal Lung and in Emphysema. **A.** Normal lung.

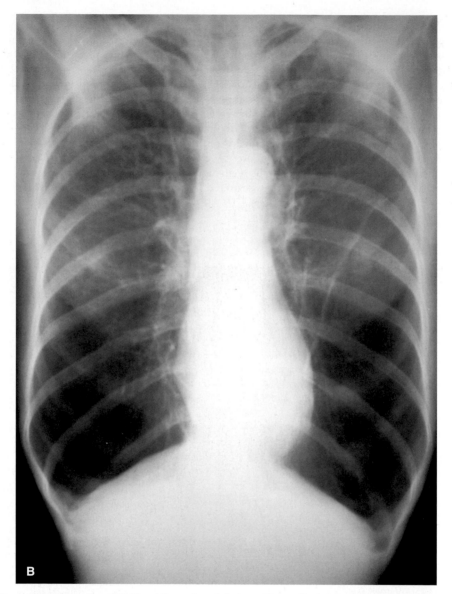

**Figure 4-8.** *(continued)* **B.** The pattern of overinflation, with low diaphragms, narrow mediastinum, and increased translucency that is seen in emphysema. The emphysema is particularly prominent in the lower regions of the lung.

## *Type B*

A typical presentation would be a man in his 50s with a history of chronic cough with expectoration for several years. This expectoration has gradually increased in severity, being present only in the winter months initially but, more recently, lasting most of the year. Acute exacerbations with frankly purulent sputum have become more common. Shortness of breath on exertion has gradually worsened, with progressively limiting exercise tolerance. The patient is almost invariably a cigarette smoker of many years' duration. This can

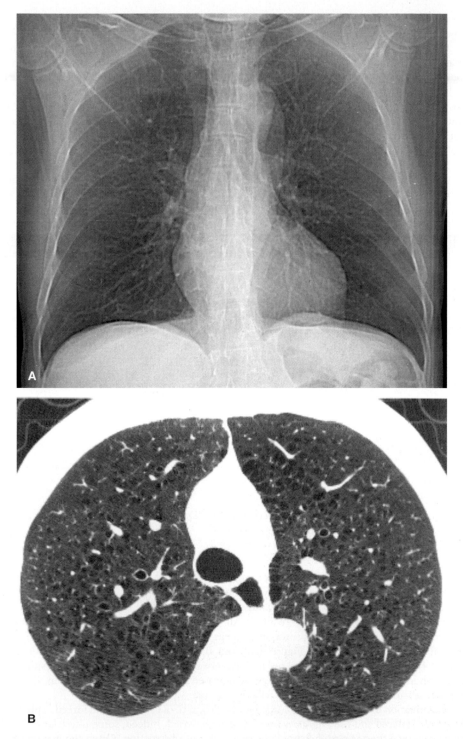

**Figure 4-9.** **A.** Appearance of normal lung using a digital technique. There is excellent resolution, and the small blood vessels can be seen. **B.** Axial section of the lungs of a patient with emphysema. Holes can be seen scattered throughout the lung. Also note the paraseptal emphysema closest to the mediastinum on the right.

be quantified as the number of cigarette packs a day multiplied by the number of years of smoking to give the "pack-years."

On examination, the patient has a stocky build with a plethoric complexion and some cyanosis. Auscultation reveals scattered rales (crackles) and rhonchi (whistles). There may be signs of fluid retention with a raised jugular venous pressure and ankle edema. The chest radiograph shows some cardiac enlargement, congested lung fields, and increased markings attributable to old infection. Parallel lines (tram lines) may be seen, probably caused by the thickened walls of inflamed bronchi. At autopsy, chronic inflammatory changes in the bronchi are the rule if the patient had severe bronchitis, but there may be severe emphysema as well. These patients are sometimes called "blue bloaters."

Some physicians believe that the essential difference between the two types is in the control of breathing. They suggest that the more severe hypoxemia and consequent higher incidence of cor pulmonale in the type B patients can be attributed to a reduced ventilatory drive, especially during sleep.

## Features of Type A and Type B Presentations in COPD

| Type A—"Pink Puffer" | Type B—"Blue Bloater" |
| --- | --- |
| Increasing dyspnea over years | Increasing dyspnea over years |
| Little or no cough | Frequent cough with sputum |
| Marked chest overexpansion | Moderate or no increase in chest volume |
| No cyanosis | Often cyanosis |
| Quiet breath sounds | Rales and rhonchi |
| Normal jugular venous pressure | Raised jugular venous pressure |
| No peripheral edema | Peripheral edema |
| Arterial $P_{O_2}$ only moderately depressed | $P_{O_2}$ often very low |
| Arterial $P_{CO_2}$ normal | $P_{CO_2}$ often raised |

## Pulmonary Function

Most of the features of disordered function in COPD follow from the pathologic features discussed earlier and illustrated in Figures 4-2 to 4-7.

### Ventilatory Capacity and Mechanics

The forced expiratory volume in 1 second ($FEV_1$), forced vital capacity (FVC), forced expiratory volume as a percentage of vital capacity (FEV/FVC%), forced expiratory flow ($FEF_{25-75\%}$), and maximum expiratory flow at 50% and 75% of exhaled vital capacity ($\dot{V}max_{50\%}$ and $\dot{V}max_{75\%}$) are all reduced. All of these measurements reflect the airway obstruction, whether caused by excessive mucus in the lumen or thickening of the wall by inflammatory changes (see Figure 4.1A and B) or by the loss of radial traction (see Figure 4-1C). The FVC is reduced because the airways close prematurely during expiration at an abnormally high lung volume, giving an increased residual volume (RV). Again, all three mechanisms of Figure 4-1 may be contributing factors.

Examination of the spirogram shows that the flow rate over most of the forced expiration is greatly reduced and the *expiratory time* is much increased. Indeed, some physicians regard this prolonged time as a useful simple bedside index of obstruction. Often the maneuver is terminated by breathlessness when the patient is still exhaling. The low flow rate over most of the forced expiration partly reflects the reduced elastic recoil of the emphysematous lung, which generates the pressure responsible for flow under these conditions of dynamic compression (see Figure 1-6). Typically, the $FEV_1$ may be reduced to less than 0.8 liters in severe disease (normal value is approximately 4 liters in young healthy males). Note that the normal values depend on age, height, and gender (see Appendix A).

In some patients, the $FEV_1$, FVC, and FEV/FVC% may increase significantly after the administration of a bronchodilator aerosol (e.g., 0.5% albuterol by nebulizer for 3 minutes). Such reactive airways are particularly likely to be found in a patient with bronchitis during an exacerbation of infection. Significant response to bronchodilators over a period of weeks suggests asthma, and this disease may overlap with chronic bronchitis (asthmatic bronchitis). Some physicians give bronchodilators to all patients with COPD.

The expiratory flow–volume curve is grossly abnormal in severe disease. Figure 1-8 shows that, after a brief interval of moderately high flow, flow is strikingly reduced as the airways collapse, and flow limitation by dynamic compression occurs. The graphed curve often has a scooped-out appearance. Flow is greatly reduced in relation to lung volume and ceases at a high lung volume because of premature airway closure (see Figure 1-5B). However, the inspiratory flow–volume curve may be normal or nearly so (see Figure 1-9).

The total lung capacity (TLC), functional residual capacity (FRC), and RV are all typically increased in emphysema. Often, the RV/TLC% may exceed 40% (less than 30% in young healthy patients). There is often a striking discrepancy between the FRC determined by the body plethysmograph and by the gas dilution techniques (helium equilibration), the former being higher by 1 liter or more. This may be caused by regions of uncommunicating lung behind grossly distorted airways. However, the disparity more often reflects the slow equilibration process in poorly ventilated areas. These static lung volumes are also often abnormal in patients with chronic bronchitis, although the increases in volume are generally less marked.

Elastic recoil of the lung is reduced in emphysema (see Figure 3-1), the pressure–volume curve being displaced up and to the left. This change reflects the disorganization and loss of elastic tissue as a result of the destruction of alveolar walls. The transpulmonary pressure at TLC is low. In uncomplicated chronic bronchitis in the absence of emphysema, the pressure–volume curve may be nearly normal because the parenchyma is little affected.

Airway resistance (related to lung volume) is increased in COPD. All the factors shown in Figure 4-1 may be responsible. However, it is possible to distinguish between an increased resistance caused by intrinsic narrowing of the airway or debris in the lumen (Figure 4-1A and B) and the loss of elastic recoil and radial traction (Figure 4-1C). This can be done by relating resistance to the static elastic recoil (compare Figure 1-10).

Figure 4-10 shows airway conductance (reciprocal of resistance) plotted against static transpulmonary pressure in a series of 10 healthy patients, 10 patients with emphysema (without bronchitis), and 10 asthmatics. The measurements were made during a quiet, unforced expiration. Note that the relationship between conductance and transpulmonary pressure for the patients with emphysema was almost normal. In other words, we can ascribe their reduced ventilatory capacity almost entirely to the effects of the smaller elastic recoil pressure of the lung. This not only reduces the effective driving pressure during a forced expiration but also allows the airways to collapse more easily because of the loss of radial traction. The small displacement of the emphysematous line to the right probably reflects the distortion and loss of airways in this disease.

By contrast, the line for the asthmatics shows that the airway conductance was greatly reduced at a given recoil pressure. Thus, the higher resistance in these patients can be ascribed to intrinsic narrowing of the airways caused by contraction of smooth muscle and inflammatory changes in the airways. After inhalation of a bronchodilator drug, isoproterenol, the asthmatic line moved toward the normal position (not shown in Figure 4-10).

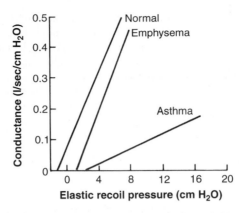

**Figure 4-10. Relationships Between Airway Conductance and Elastic Recoil Pressure in Obstructive Pulmonary Disease.** Note that the line for emphysema lies close to the normal line. It is evident that any increase in airway resistance is chiefly caused by the smaller elastic recoil of the lung. By contrast, in asthma, the line is markedly abnormal due to the intrinsic narrowing of the airways. (From Colebatch HJH, Finucane KE, Smith MM. Pulmonary conductance and elastic recoil relationships in asthma and emphysema. *J Appl Physiol* 1973;34:143–153.)

Comparable data are not available for a group of patients with chronic bronchitis without emphysema because it is virtually impossible to select such a group during life. However, Figure 4-10 clarifies the behavior of different types of airway obstruction.

## *Gas Exchange*

Ventilation–perfusion inequality is inevitable in COPD and leads to hypoxemia with or without $CO_2$ retention. Typically, the type A patient has only moderate hypoxemia ($P_{O_2}$ often in the high 60s or 70s), and the arterial $P_{CO_2}$ is normal. By contrast, the type B patient often has severe hypoxemia ($P_{O_2}$ often in the 50s or 40s) with an increased $P_{CO_2}$, especially in advanced disease.

The alveolar–arterial difference for $P_{O_2}$ is always increased, especially in patients with severe bronchitis. An analysis based on the concept of the ideal point (see Figure 2-7) reveals increases in both physiologic dead space and physiologic shunt. The dead space is particularly increased in emphysema, whereas high values for physiologic shunt are especially common in bronchitis.

The reasons for these differences are clarified by the results obtained with the inert gas elimination technique. First, review Figure 2-8, which shows a typical pattern in a normal subject. By contrast, Figure 4-11 shows a typical distribution in a patient with advanced type A disease. This 76-year-old man had a history of increasing dyspnea over several years. The chest radiograph showed hyperinflation with attenuated small pulmonary vessels. The arterial $P_{O_2}$ and $P_{CO_2}$ were 68 and 39 mm Hg, respectively.

The distribution shows that a large amount of ventilation went to lung units with high ventilation–perfusion ratios ($V_A/Q$) (compare Figure 2-8). This would be shown as physiologic dead space in the ideal point analysis, and the excessive ventilation is largely wasted from the point of view of gas exchange. By contrast, there is little blood flow to units with an abnormally low $V_A/Q$. This explains the relatively mild degree of hypoxemia in the patient and the fact that the calculated physiologic shunt was only slightly increased.

These findings can be contrasted with those shown in Figure 4-12, which shows the distribution in a 47-year-old man with advanced chronic bronchitis and type B disease. He was a heavy smoker and had had a productive cough for many years. The arterial $P_{O_2}$ and $P_{CO_2}$ were 47 and 50 mm Hg, respectively. Note that there was some increase in ventilation to high

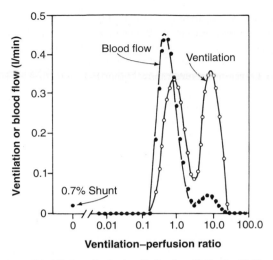

**Figure 4-11. Distribution of Ventilation–Perfusion Ratios in a Patient with Type A COPD.** Note the large amount of ventilation to units with high ventilation–perfusion ratios (physiologic dead space). (From Wagner PD, Dantzker DR, Dueck R, et al. Ventilation–perfusion inequality in chronic pulmonary disease. *J Clin Invest* 1977;59:203–206.)

$\dot{V}_A/\dot{Q}$ units (physiologic dead space). However, the distribution chiefly shows large amounts of blood flow to low $\dot{V}_A/\dot{Q}$ units (physiologic shunt), accounting for his severe hypoxemia. It is remarkable that there was no blood flow to unventilated alveoli (true shunt). Indeed, true shunts of more than a few percent are uncommon in COPD. Note that although the patterns shown in Figures 4-11 and 4-12 are typical, considerable variation is seen in patients with COPD.

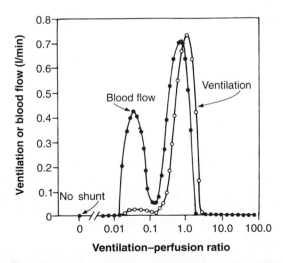

**Figure 4-12. Distribution of Ventilation–Perfusion Ratios in a Patient with Type B COPD.** There is a large amount of blood flow to units with low ventilation–perfusion ratios (physiologic shunt). (From Wagner PD, Dantzker DR, Dueck R, et al. Ventilation–perfusion inequality in chronic pulmonary disease. *J Clin Invest* 1977;59:203–206.)

On exercise, the arterial $P_{O_2}$ may fall or rise. The changes depend on the response of the ventilation and the cardiac output and the changes in the distribution of ventilation and blood flow. In some patients at least, the main factor in the fall of $P_{O_2}$ is the limited cardiac output, which, in the presence of ventilation–perfusion inequality, exaggerates any hypoxemia. Patients with $CO_2$ retention often show higher $P_{CO_2}$ values on exercise because of their limited ventilatory response.

The reasons for the ventilation–perfusion inequality are clear when we consider the disorganization of the lung architecture in emphysema (Figures 4-2 and 4-3) and the abnormalities in airways in chronic bronchitis (Figure 4-6). There is ample evidence of uneven ventilation as determined by the single-breath nitrogen washout (see Figure 1-10). In addition, topographic measurements with radioactive materials show regional inequality of both ventilation and blood flow. The blood flow inequality is largely caused by the destruction of portions of the capillary bed.

The deleterious effects of airway obstruction on gas exchange are reduced by collateral ventilation that occurs in these patients. Communicating channels normally exist between adjacent alveoli and between neighboring small airways, and there have been many experimental demonstrations of these. The fact that there is so little blood flow to unventilated units in these patients (Figures 4-11 and 4-12) emphasizes the effectiveness of collateral ventilation because some airways must presumably be completely obstructed, especially in severe bronchitis (see Figure 1-12).

Another factor that reduces the amount of ventilation–perfusion inequality is hypoxic vasoconstriction. (See *Respiratory Physiology: The Essentials*, 9th ed., p. 50.) This local response to a low alveolar $P_{O_2}$ reduces the blood flow to poorly ventilated and unventilated regions, minimizing the arterial hypoxemia. When patients with COPD are given bronchodilators, for example, albuterol, they sometimes develop a slight fall in arterial $P_{O_2}$. This is probably caused by the vasodilator action of these β-adrenergic drugs, increasing the blood flow to poorly ventilated areas. This finding is more marked in asthma (see Figures 4-17 and 4-18).

The arterial $P_{CO_2}$ is often normal in patients with mild to moderate COPD despite their ventilation–perfusion inequality. Any tendency for the arterial $P_{CO_2}$ to rise stimulates the chemoreceptors, thus increasing ventilation to the alveoli (see Figure 2-9). As disease becomes more severe, the arterial $P_{CO_2}$ may rise. This is particularly likely to occur in type B patients. The increased work of breathing is an important factor, but there is also evidence that the sensitivity of the respiratory center to $CO_2$ is reduced in some of these patients.

If the arterial $P_{CO_2}$ rises, the pH tends to fall, resulting in respiratory acidosis. In some patients, the $P_{CO_2}$ rises so slowly that the kidney is able to compensate adequately by retaining bicarbonate, and the pH remains almost constant (compensated respiratory acidosis). In other instances, the $P_{CO_2}$ rises more suddenly, perhaps as a consequence of an acute chest infection. Under these conditions, acute respiratory acidosis may occur (see Chapter 8, Respiratory Failure).

Additional information about gas exchange in these patients can be obtained by measuring the diffusing capacity (transfer factor) for carbon monoxide (see Figure 2-11). The diffusing capacity as measured by the single-breath method is particularly likely to be reduced in patients with severe emphysema. By contrast, patients with chronic bronchitis but little parenchymal destruction may have normal values.

## Pulmonary Circulation

The pulmonary artery pressure frequently rises in patients with COPD as their disease progresses. Several factors are responsible. In emphysema, large portions of the capillary bed are destroyed, thus increasing vascular resistance. Hypoxic vasoconstriction also raises the pulmonary arterial pressure, and often an exacerbation of chest infection causes an additional transient increase as the hypoxia worsens. Acidosis may exaggerate the hypoxic vasoconstriction. In advanced disease, histologic changes in the walls of the small arteries occur. Finally, these patients often develop polycythemia as a response to the hypoxemia, thus increasing blood viscosity. This occurs most commonly in patients with severe bronchitis, who tend to have the lowest arterial $P_{O_2}$.

Fluid retention with dependent edema and engorged neck veins may occur, especially in type B patients. The right heart often enlarges with characteristic radiologic and electrocardiographic appearances. The term "cor pulmonale" is given to this condition, but whether it should be regarded as right heart failure is disputed. The output of the heart is normally increased because it is operating high on the Starling curve, and the output can rise further on exercise.

## Control of Ventilation

As indicated previously, some patients with COPD, particularly those with severe chronic bronchitis, develop $CO_2$ retention because they do not sufficiently increase the ventilation to their alveoli. The reasons why some patients behave in this way and some do not are not completely understood. One factor is the increased work of breathing as a result of the high airway resistance. As a consequence, the $O_2$ cost of breathing may be enormous (Figure 4-13). Normal subjects have an abnormally small ventilatory response to inhaled $CO_2$ if they are asked to breathe through a high resistance. Thus, a patient with a severely limited $O_2$ consumption may be willing to forgo a normal arterial $P_{CO_2}$ to obtain the advantage of a reduced work of breathing and a correspondingly reduced $O_2$ cost. However, the correlation between airway resistance and arterial $P_{CO_2}$ is sufficiently poor that some other factor must be involved.

Measurements of the ventilatory response to inhaled $CO_2$ show that there are significant differences among normal subjects. These differences are partly caused by genetic factors. Some patients have a reduced respiratory center output in response to inhaled $CO_2$, many have a mechanical obstruction to ventilation, and some patients have both. Thus, it is possible that the ventilatory response of a patient in the face of severe ventilation–perfusion inequality and increased work of breathing is predetermined to some extent by these factors.

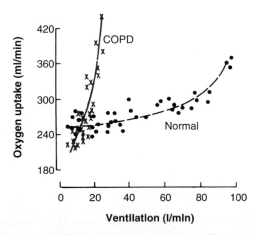

**Figure 4-13. Oxygen Uptake During Voluntary Hyperventilation in Patients with COPD.** Note the high values compared with those of the normal subjects. (From Cherniack RM, Cherniack L, Naimark A. *Respiration in Health and Disease.* 2nd ed. Philadelphia, PA: WB Saunders, 1972.)

## Changes in Early Disease

So far we have been concerned mainly with pulmonary function in patients with well-established disease. However, relatively little can be done to reverse the disease process in this group, and the treatment is limited chiefly to prevention and control of infection, relief of bronchoconstriction, and general rehabilitative measures. Rehabilitation programs can definitely improve a patient's quality of life in spite of the fact that the pathological changes may not be reversed. There is a great deal of interest in identifying patients with early disease in the hope that the changes can be arrested or reversed. At the very least, these patients could be strongly advised to stop smoking.

It was emphasized in Chapter 1 that because relatively little of the airway resistance resides in small airways (less than 2 mm wide), pathophysiologic changes there may go unnoticed by the usual function tests. There is some evidence that the earliest changes in COPD occur in these small airways. Tests of small airway function that are currently being assessed include the $FEV_1$, $FEF_{25-75\%}$, $\dot{V}max_{50\%}$, $\dot{V}max_{75\%}$, and closing volume. The practical value of these tests for the early detection of disease is still uncertain.

## Treatment of Patients with COPD

It is critically important that the patient stops smoking, but often this is difficult to achieve. Exposure to occupational and atmospheric pollution should be reduced as far as possible. Chronic bronchitis should be treated with antibiotics and also with bronchodilators if there is a reversible element. Some physicians recommend bronchodilators for all patients. Rehabilitation is helpful in advanced disease.

## Lung Volume Reduction Surgery

Surgery to reduce the volume of the overexpanded lung can be valuable in selected cases. The physiologic basis is that reducing the volume increases the radial traction on the airways and therefore helps to limit dynamic compression. In addition, the inspiratory muscles, particularly the diaphragm, are shortened with consequent improvement in their mechanical efficiency. Initially, the emphasis was on resecting bullae, but now good results can be obtained in patients with more diffuse emphysema. The aim is to remove emphysematous and avascular areas and to preserve the nearly normal regions. Criteria for surgery usually include an $FEV_1$ of less than about one-third of predicted; heterogeneity of emphysema demonstrated by computed demography and scanning; large RV, FRC, and TLC, and an arterial less than about 55 mm Hg. Significant improvements in pulmonary function test and perceived quality of life can be expected for at least 1 year in many cases.

---

## ▶ Asthma

*This disease is characterized by increased responsiveness of the airways to various stimuli and is manifested by inflammation and widespread narrowing of the airways that changes in severity, either spontaneously or as a result of treatment.*

## Pathology

The airways have hypertrophied smooth muscle that contracts during an attack, causing bronchoconstriction (Figure 4-1B). In addition, there is hypertrophy of mucous glands, edema of the bronchial wall, and extensive infiltration by eosinophils and lymphocytes (Figure 4-14). The mucus is increased and is also abnormal; it is thick, tenacious, and slow moving. In severe cases, many airways are occluded by mucous plugs, some of which may be coughed up in the sputum. The sputum typically is scant and white. Subepithelial fibrosis

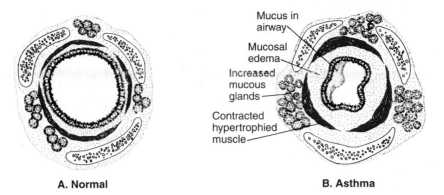

**A. Normal**    **B. Asthma**

Mucus in airway
Mucosal edema
Increased mucous glands
Contracted hypertrophied muscle

**Figure 4-14. Bronchial Wall in Asthma (Diagrammatic).** Note the hypertrophied, contracted smooth muscle, edema, mucous gland hypertrophy, and secretion in the lumen.

is common in patients with chronic asthma and is part of the process called remodeling. In uncomplicated asthma, there is no destruction of alveolar walls and there are no copious purulent bronchial secretions. Occasionally, the abundance of eosinophils in the sputum gives a purulent appearance, which may be wrongly ascribed to infection.

## Pathogenesis

Rapid progress is being made in this area, and the following account will no doubt be modified. Two features that appear to be common to all asthmatics are airway hyperresponsiveness and airway inflammation. Research suggests that the hyperresponsiveness is a consequence of the inflammation, and some investigators believe that airway inflammation is responsible for all the associated features of asthma, including the increased airway responsiveness, airway edema, hypersecretion of mucus, and inflammatory cell infiltration. However, a fundamental abnormality of airway smooth muscle or regulation of airway tone is possible in some patients.

Epidemiologic studies indicate that asthma begins in childhood in the majority of cases and that an allergic diathesis often plays an important role. However, environmental factors appear to be important and may be responsible for the increase in the prevalence and severity of asthma over the last 20 to 40 years in modernized, affluent western countries. Frequent exposure to typical childhood infections and environments favoring fecal contamination are associated with a lower incidence of asthma. These observations and others have led to the "hygiene hypothesis," which suggests that children in a critical stage of development of the immune response who are not frequently exposed to typical childhood infectious agents may more frequently develop an allergic diathesis and asthma. Other hypotheses have also been proposed to explain the increases in prevalence including obesity, poor physical fitness, and exposure to pollutants.

The trigger for the development of airway inflammation cannot always be identified. It is well recognized in some instances, as in the case for some antigens in persons with allergic asthma (Figure 4-15). However, in other types of asthma, such as exercise-induced asthma or asthma following a viral respiratory tract infection, the trigger is not recognized. Atmospheric pollutants, especially submicronic particles in automobile exhaust gases, may also play a role.

A single inflammatory cell type or inflammatory mediator does not appear to be responsible for all manifestations of asthma. Eosinophils, mast cells, neutrophils, macrophages, and basophils have all been implicated. There is also evidence that noninflammatory cells, including airway epithelial cells and neural cells, especially those of peptidergic nerves,

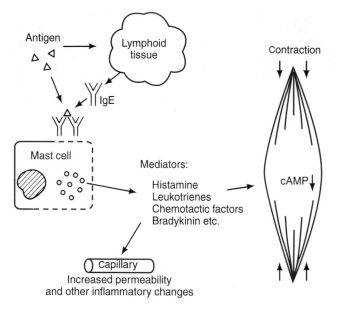

**Figure 4-15. Some Pathogenic Changes in Allergic Asthma.** (See text for details.)

contribute to the inflammation. Some investigators believe that eosinophils play a central effector role in most cases of asthma. There is also evidence that lymphocytes, especially T-cells, are implicated, both because they respond to specific antigens and because they have a role as a modulator of inflammatory cell function.

Many inflammatory mediators have been identified in asthma. Cytokines are probably important, particularly those associated with Th-2, helper T-cell activation. These cytokines include interleukin-3, IL-4, IL-5, and IL-13. It is believed that these cytokines are at least partly responsible for modulating inflammatory and immune cell function and for supporting the inflammatory response in the airway. Other inflammatory mediators that probably play a role, particularly in acute bronchoconstriction, include arachidonic acid metabolites, such as leukotrienes and prostaglandins, platelet-activating factor (PAF), neuropeptides, reactive oxygen species, kinins, histamine, and adenosine.

Asthma also has a genetic component. Population studies show that it is a complex genetic disorder with both environmental and genetic components. The latter is not a single gene trait but is polygenic. Associations of asthma with a variety of chromosomal loci through linkage analysis have been demonstrated.

## Clinical Features

Asthma commonly begins in children but may occur at any age. The patient may have a previous history to suggest atopy, including allergic rhinitis, eczema, or urticaria, and may relate asthmatic attacks to a specific allergen, for example, ragweed or cats. Such a patient is said to have allergic asthma. Many such patients have an increased total serum IgE, increased specific IgE, and peripheral blood eosinophils. If there is no general history of allergy and no external allergen can be identified, the term "nonallergic asthma" is used.

In all asthmatics, there is general hyperreactivity of the airways, with the result that nonspecific irritants, such as smoke, cold air, and exercise, cause symptoms. The hyperreactivity (or hyperresponsiveness) of the airways can be tested by exposing the patient to increasing inhaled concentrations of methacholine or histamine and measuring the $FEV_1$ (or airway resistance). The concentration that results in a 20% fall in $FEV_1$ is known as the $PC_{20}$ (provocative concentration 20).

Attacks may follow exercise, especially in a cold environment. Aspirin ingestion is a cause in some individuals because of inhibition of the cyclooxygenase pathway. This may have a genetic component. Between attacks, the patient may have no symptoms, although inflammation persists. Psychological factors are important.

During an attack, the patient may be extremely dyspneic, orthopneic, and anxious. The accessory muscles of respiration are active. The lungs are hyperinflated, and musical rhonchi are heard in all areas. The pulse is rapid, and pulsus paradoxicus may be present (marked fall in systolic and pulse pressure during inspiration). The sputum is scant and viscid. The chest radiograph reveals hyperinflation but is otherwise normal.

*Status asthmaticus* refers to an attack that continues for hours or even days without remission despite bronchodilator therapy. There are often signs of exhaustion, dehydration, and marked tachycardia. The chest may become ominously silent, and vigorous treatment is urgently required.

## Bronchoactive Drugs

Drugs that reverse or prevent bronchoconstriction play a major role in the treatment of patients with asthma. They are also useful in patients with chronic bronchitis who have some reversible airway obstruction.

### β-Adrenergic Agonists

β-Adrenergic receptors are of two types: $\beta_1$ receptors exist in the heart and elsewhere, and their stimulation increases heart rate and the force of contraction of cardiac muscle. Stimulation of $\beta_2$ receptors relaxes smooth muscle in the bronchi, blood vessels, and uterus. Partially or completely $\beta_2$-selective adrenergic agonists have now completely replaced nonselective agonists. Available drugs include metaproterenol, albuterol, terbutaline, and pirbuterol. These agents have an intermediate duration of action. Long-acting agents, such as formoterol and salmeterol, are also available but should always be used in combination with inhaled corticosteroids. All these drugs bind to $\beta_2$ receptors in the lung and directly relax airway smooth muscle by increasing the activity of adenyl cyclase. This in turn raises the concentration of intracellular cAMP, which is reduced in an asthma attack (Fig. 4-14). They also have effects on airway edema and airway inflammation. Their anti-inflammatory effects are mediated by direct inhibition of inflammatory cell function via binding to $\beta_2$ receptors on the cell surface. There is some polymorphism in these receptors that affects the responses.

These drugs are delivered by aerosol, preferably using a metered-dose inhaler or a nebulizer. In the past, there was concern about possible tachyphylaxis, particularly in the drug's ability to reverse induced bronchoconstriction when used regularly. However, this is now less of an issue.

### Inhaled Corticosteroids

Corticosteroids appear to have two separate functions: they inhibit the inflammatory/immune response, and they enhance β receptor expression or function. Inhaled corticosteroids are now increasingly used to treat patients with asthma. Some physicians believe that all patients with asthma benefit from inhaled corticosteroids. However, other physicians feel that patients whose disease is controlled easily with intermittent $\beta_2$ agonists or a symptom-based treatment plan do not require corticosteroids. Current guidelines recommend corticosteroid use in asthmatics who use β agonists more than twice a week. A wide variety of inhaled corticosteroids are now available, and when used as directed, result in minimal systemic absorption of corticosteroid with almost no serious side effects.

## Bronchoactive Drugs for Asthma

*β-Adrenergic Agonists*
Selective $β_2$ types are now exclusively used.
Long-acting forms are useful in prolonged management especially in conjunction with inhaled corticosteroids.
Short-acting forms are reserved for rescue.

*Inhaled Corticosteroids*
These are given by aerosol and are often indicated except in the mildest cases of asthma.

*Auxiliary Drugs*
Antileukotrienes, methylxanthine, and cromolyn may be useful adjuncts.

## Methylxanthines

The mechanism of action of methylxanthines, including theophylline and aminophylline, is uncertain. They have modest anti-inflammatory properties and are also bronchodilators, although only about one-fourth as potent as $β_2$ agonists. Measurement of blood levels is an aid to developing the correct dose and avoiding side effects.

## Anticholinergics

There is evidence that the parasympathetic nervous system may play a part in the asthma reaction. However, anticholinergics have only a modest bronchodilating effect and only in a subset of patients with asthma. By contrast, patients with COPD with reversible bronchoconstriction respond more consistently, and anticholinergics are useful here.

## Cromolyn and Nedocromil

Although these two drugs are structurally unrelated, they apparently have similar mechanisms of action. They were originally thought to be mast cell stabilizers (Figure 4.15), but it is now recognized that they have broad-ranging effects. They are not direct bronchodilators but presumably work by blocking airway inflammation.

## New Therapies

Leukotriene receptor antagonists and 5-lipoxygenase inhibitors are available, but their role in clinical asthma therapy is still being clarified. To avoid glucocorticoids, they are often used in children and may be of particular benefit to patients whose asthma is exacerbated by aspirin and other nonsteroidal anti-inflammatory drugs. There is some evidence that receptor antagonists are valuable in severe, persistent asthma. Another recently introduced drug is Omalizumab, which is a monoclonal antibody to IgE and can be a potent steroid sparring agent. However, it is expensive.

# Pulmonary Function

As was the case with chronic bronchitis and emphysema, the changes in lung function generally follow clearly from the pathology of asthma.

## Ventilatory Capacity and Mechanics

During an attack, all indices of expiratory flow rate are reduced significantly, including the $FEV_1$, FEV/FVC%, $FEF_{25-75\%}$, $\dot{V}max_{50\%}$, and $\dot{V}max_{75\%}$. The FVC is also usually reduced because airways close prematurely toward the end of a full expiration. Between attacks, some impairment of ventilatory capacity can usually be demonstrated, although the patient may claim to feel normal.

The response of these indices to bronchodilator drugs is of great importance in asthma (Figure 4-16). They may be tested by administering 0.5% albuterol by aerosol for 2 minutes. Typically, all indices increase substantially when a bronchodilator is administered to a patient during an attack, and the change is a valuable measure of the responsiveness of the airways. The extent of the increase varies according to the severity of the disease. In status asthmaticus, little change may be seen because the bronchi have become unresponsive. Again, patients in remission may show only minor improvement, although generally there is some.

There is some evidence that the relative change in $FEV_1$ and FVC after bronchodilator therapy indicates whether the bronchospasm has been completely relieved. During an asthma attack, both the $FEV_1$ and FVC tend to increase by the same fraction, with the result that the FEV/FVC% remains low and almost constant. However, when the tone of the airway muscle is nearly normal, the $FEV_1$ responds more than the FVC, and the FEV/FVC% approaches the normal value of approximately 75%.

The flow–volume curve in asthma has the typical obstructive pattern, although it may not exhibit the scooped-out appearance seen in emphysema (see Figure 1-8). After a bronchodilator, flows are higher at all lung volumes, and the whole curve may shift as the TLC and RV are reduced.

Static lung volumes are increased, and remarkably high values for FRC and TLC during asthma attacks have been reported. The increased RV is caused by premature airway closure during a full expiration as a result of the increased smooth muscle tone, edema and inflammation of the airway walls, and abnormal secretions. The cause of the increased FRC and TLC is not fully understood. However, there is some loss of elastic recoil, and the pressure–volume curve is shifted upward and to the left (see Figure 3-1). This tends to return toward normal after a bronchodilator has been given. There is some evidence that changes in the surface tension of the alveolar lining layer may be responsible for the altered elastic properties. The rise in lung volume tends to decrease resistance of the airways by increasing their radial traction. The FRC measured by helium dilution is usually considerably below that found with the body plethysmograph, reflecting the presence of occluded airways or the delayed equilibration of poorly ventilated areas.

Airway resistance as measured in the body plethysmograph is raised, and it falls after a bronchodilator. It is likely that the bronchospasm affects airways of all sizes, and the relationship between airway conductance and elastic recoil pressure is significantly abnormal (Figure 4-10). Narrowing of the large- and medium-sized bronchi can be seen directly at bronchoscopy.

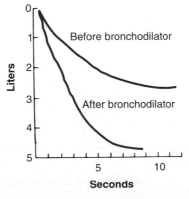

**Figure 4-16. Examples of Forced Expirations Before and After Bronchodilator Therapy in a Patient with Bronchial Asthma.** Note the striking increase in flow rate and vital capacity. (From Bates DV, Macklem PT, and Christie RV. *Respiratory Function in Disease.* 2nd ed. Philadelphia, PA: WB Saunders, 1971.)

## Gas Exchange

Arterial hypoxemia is common in asthma and is caused by ventilation–perfusion ($\dot{V}_A/Q$) inequality. There is ample evidence of uneven ventilation, and measurements with radioactive gases show regions of reduced ventilation. Marked topographical inequality of blood flow is also seen, and, typically, different areas show transient reductions at different times. Both physiologic dead space and physiologic shunt are generally abnormally high.

An example of a distribution of ventilation–perfusion ratios in a 47-year-old asthmatic is shown in Figure 4-17. This patient had only mild symptoms at the time of the measurement. The distribution is strikingly different from the normal distribution shown in Figure 2-8. Note especially the bimodal distribution with a considerable amount of the total blood flow (approximately 25%) to units with a low $\dot{V}_A/Q$ (approximately 0.1). This accounts for the patient's mild hypoxemia, the arterial $P_{O_2}$ being 81 mm Hg. There is no pure shunt (blood flow to unventilated alveoli), a surprising finding in view of the mucous plugging of airways, which is a feature of the disease.

When this patient was given the bronchodilator isoproterenol by aerosol, there was an increase in $FEF_{25-75\%}$ from 3.4 to 4.2 liters/s. Thus, there was some relief of his bronchospasm. The changes in the distribution of ventilation–perfusion ratios are shown in Figure 4-18. Note that the blood flow to the low $\dot{V}_A/Q$ alveoli increased from approximately 25 to 50% of the flow, resulting in a fall in arterial $P_{O_2}$ from 81 to 70 mm Hg. The mean $\dot{V}_A/Q$ of the low mode increased slightly from 0.10 to 0.14, indicating that the ventilation to these units increased slightly more than their blood flow. Again no shunt was seen.

Many bronchodilators, including isoproterenol, aminophylline, and terbutaline, decrease the arterial $P_{O_2}$ in asthmatics. The mechanism of the increased hypoxemia is apparently relief of vasoconstriction in poorly ventilated areas. This vasoconstriction probably results from the release of mediators, like the bronchoconstriction. The fall in $P_{O_2}$ is accompanied by increases in physiologic shunt and dead space. However, in practice, the favorable effects of the drugs on airway resistance far exceed the disadvantages of the mild additional hypoxemia.

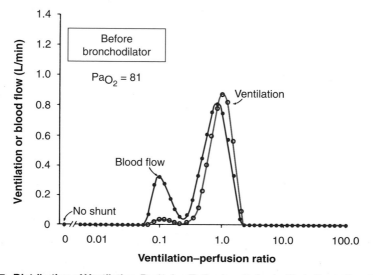

**Figure 4-17. Distribution of Ventilation–Perfusion Ratios in a Patient with Asthma.** Note the bimodal appearance, with approximately 25% of the blood flowing to units with ventilation–perfusion ratios in the region of 0.1.

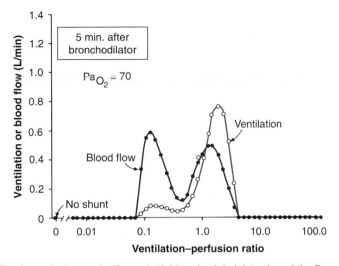

**Figure 4-18. The Same Patient as in Figure 4-16 After the Administration of the Bronchodilator Isoproterenol by Aerosol.** Note the increase in blood flow to the units with low ventilation–perfusion ratios and the corresponding fall in arterial $P_{O_2}$.

The absence of shunt—that is, blood flow to unventilated lung units—in Figures 4-17 and 4-18 is striking, especially because asthmatics who come to autopsy have mucous plugs in many of their airways. Presumably, the explanation is collateral ventilation that reaches lung situated behind completely closed bronchioles. This is shown diagrammatically in Figure 1-11. The same mechanism probably exists in the lungs of patients with chronic bronchitis (see for example, Figure 4-12).

The arterial $P_{CO_2}$ in patients with asthma is typically normal or low, at least until late in the disease. The $P_{CO_2}$ is prevented from rising by increased ventilation to the alveoli in the face of the ventilation–perfusion inequality (compare Figure 2-9). In many patients, the $P_{CO_2}$ may be in the middle or low 30s, possibly as a result of stimulation of the peripheral chemoreceptors by the mild hypoxemia or stimulation of intrapulmonary receptors.

In status asthmaticus, the arterial $P_{CO_2}$ may begin to rise and the pH to fall. This is an ominous development that denotes impending respiratory failure and signals the need for urgent and intensive treatment. Mechanical ventilation may be necessary (see Chapter 10). Deaths from asthma have apparently increased in recent years, and respiratory failure is one cause. Another cause may be overuse of β-adrenergic drugs via inhalers. However, some severe asthmatics are undertreated because the dangers of their disease are not appreciated sufficiently.

The diffusing capacity for carbon monoxide is typically normal or high in uncomplicated asthma. If it is reduced, associated emphysema should be suspected. The reason for the increased diffusing capacity is probably the large lung volume. Hyperinflation increases the diffusing capacity in normal subjects, presumably by increasing the area of the blood–gas interface.

## ▶ Localized Airway Obstruction

So far, this chapter has been devoted to generalized airway obstruction, both irreversible, as in emphysema and chronic bronchitis, and reversible, as in asthma. (Some chronic bronchitis may show some reversibility.) Localized obstruction is less common and generally causes less functional impairment. Obstruction may be within the lumen of the airway, in the wall, or as a result of compression from outside the wall (Figure 4-1).

# Tracheal Obstruction

This can be caused by an inhaled foreign body; stenosis after the use of an indwelling trache-ostomy tube; or compressing masses, such as an enlarged thyroid. There is inspiratory and expiratory stridor, abnormal inspiratory and expiratory flow–volume curves (see Figure 1-9), and no response to bronchodilators. Hypoventilation may result in hypercapnia and hypox-emia (see Figure 2-2).

# Bronchial Obstruction

This is often caused by a foreign body, for example, an inhaled peanut. The right lung is more frequently affected than the left because the left main bronchus makes a sharper angle with the trachea than does the right. Other common causes are bronchial tumors, either malignant or benign, and compression of a bronchus by enlarged surrounding lymph nodes. This last cause particularly affects the right middle lobe bronchus because of its anatomic relationships.

If obstruction is complete, absorption atelectasis occurs because the sum of the partial pressures in mixed venous blood is less than that in alveolar gas. (See *Respiratory Physiology: The Essentials*, 9th ed., p. 158). The collapsed lobe is often visible on the radiograph, and compensatory overinflation of adjacent lung and displacement of a fissure may also be seen. Perfusion of the unventilated lung is reduced because of hypoxic vasoconstriction and also the increased vascular resistance caused by the mechanical effects of the reduced volume on the extra-alveolar vessels and the capillaries. However, the residual blood flow contributes to hypoxemia. The most sensitive test is the alveolar–arterial $P_{O_2}$ difference during 100% $O_2$ breathing (see Figure 2-6). Infection may follow localized obstruction and lead to lung abscess. If the obstruction is in a segmental or smaller bronchus, atelectasis may not occur because of collateral ventilation (see Figure 1-11).

## KEY CONCEPTS

1. Chronic obstructive pulmonary disease is extremely common and can be very disabling. These patients have emphysema, chronic bronchitis, or a mixture of both.

2. Emphysema is a disease of the lung parenchyma characterized by the breakdown of alveolar walls with loss of lung elastic recoil and dynamic compression of airways.

3. Chronic bronchitis refers to inflammation of the airways with excessive mucus production. The lung parenchyma is normal or nearly so.

4. Asthma is characterized by increased responsiveness of the airways accompanied by inflam-mation. The airway narrowing typically varies in severity.

5. All of these diseases cause marked changes in forced expirations with reductions in the $FEV_1$, FVC, and FEV/FVC.

6. Asthma can often be treated effectively with bronchoactive drugs including β-adrenergic agonists and inhaled corticosteroids.

## QUESTIONS

1. Which form of emphysema predominantly affects the apex of the lung?
   A. That caused by $\alpha_1$-antitrypsin deficiency.
   B. Centriacinar emphysema.
   C. Panacinar emphysema.
   D. Paraseptal emphysema.
   E. Unilateral emphysema.

2. A current hypothesis for the pathogenesis of emphysema is:

    A. Damage to pulmonary capillaries by increased alveolar pressure.
    B. Chronic stimulation of bronchial mucous glands by cigarette smoking.
    C. Destruction of lung elastin and collagen by excessive action of neutrophil elastase.
    D. Excessive amounts of exercise.
    E. Hyperventilation at high altitude.

3. Alpha 1–antitrypsin deficiency:

    A. Causes severe bronchitis with emphysema.
    B. Results in emphysema at a relatively early age.
    C. Is caused by infections in early childhood.
    D. Is common in heterozygotes for the Z gene.
    E. Tends to be most marked in the upper regions of the lung.

4. Patients with COPD with the type A presentation (as opposed to type B) tend to have:

    A. More cough productive of sputum.
    B. Smaller lung volumes.
    C. Decreased lung elastic recoil.
    D. More hypoxemia.
    E. Greater tendency to develop cor pulmonale.

5. In a patient with severe bronchitis and emphysema, which of the following is likely to be normal?

    A. $FEV_1$.
    B. FVC.
    C. $FEV_1/FVC$.
    D. $FEF_{25-75\%}$.
    E. None of the above.

0. The chief mechanism of hypoxemia in patients with COPD is:

    A. Hypoventilation
    B. Diffusion impairment.
    C. Ventilation–perfusion inequality.
    D. Shunt.
    E. Abnormal hemoglobin.

7. When a bronchodilator is administered to a patient during an asthma attack, which of the following typically decreases?

    A. $FEV_1$.
    B. FEV/FVC%.
    C. FVC.
    D. $FEF_{25-75\%}$.
    E. FRC.

8. Concerning the use of β-adrenergic agonists in asthma:

    A. β1-selective agonists are preferred to β2 agonists.
    B. They relax airway smooth muscle by decreasing the concentration of adenyl cyclase.
    C. They reduce the concentration of intracellular cAMP.
    D. They reduce airway resistance.
    E. They are usually given as tablets by mouth.

# Restrictive Diseases

# 5

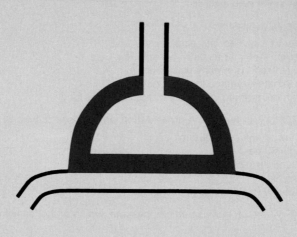

Restrictive diseases are those in which the expansion of the lung is restricted either because of alterations in the lung parenchyma, or because of disease of the pleura, the chest wall, or the neuromuscular apparatus. They are characterized by a reduced vital capacity and a small resting lung volume (usually), but the airway resistance (related to lung volume) is not increased. These diseases are therefore different from the obstructive diseases in their pure form, although mixed restrictive and obstructive conditions can occur.

## ▶ Diseases of the Lung Parenchyma

This term refers to the alveolar tissue of the lung. A brief review of the structure of this tissue is pertinent.

### Structure of the Alveolar Wall

Figure 5-1 shows an electron micrograph of a pulmonary capillary in an alveolar wall. The various structures through which oxygen passes on its way from the alveolar gas to the hemoglobin of the red blood cell are the layer of pulmonary surfactant (not shown in this preparation), alveolar epithelium, interstitium, capillary endothelium, plasma, and erythrocyte.

### Cell Types

The various cell types have different functions and different responses to injury.

#### Type 1 Epithelial Cell

This is the chief structural cell of the alveolar wall; its long protoplasmic extensions pave almost the whole alveolar surface (Figure 5-1). The main function of this cell is mechanical support. It rarely divides and is not very active metabolically. When type 1 cells are injured, they are replaced by type 2 cells, which later transform into type 1 cells.

#### Type 2 Epithelial Cell

This is a nearly globular cell (Figure 5-2) that gives little structural support to the alveolar wall but is metabolically active. The electron micrograph shows the lamellated bodies that contain phospholipids. This is formed in the endoplasmic reticulum, passed through the Golgi apparatus, and eventually extruded into the alveolar space to form surfactant. (See *Respiratory Physiology: The Essentials*, 9th ed., p. 105). After injury to the alveolar wall, these cells rapidly divide to line the surface and then later transform into type 1 cells. A type 3 cell has also been described, but it is rare and its function is unknown.

#### Alveolar Macrophage

This scavenger cell roams around the alveolar wall phagocytosing foreign particles and bacteria. The cell contains lysozymes that digest engulfed foreign matter.

#### Fibroblast

This cell synthesizes collagen and elastin, which are components of the interstitium of the alveolar wall. After various disease insults, large amounts of these materials may be laid down. This results in interstitial fibrosis.

### Interstitium

This fills the space between the alveolar epithelium and the capillary endothelium. Figure 5-1 shows that it is thin on one side of the capillary, where it consists only of the fused basement membranes of the epithelial and endothelial layers. On the other side of the

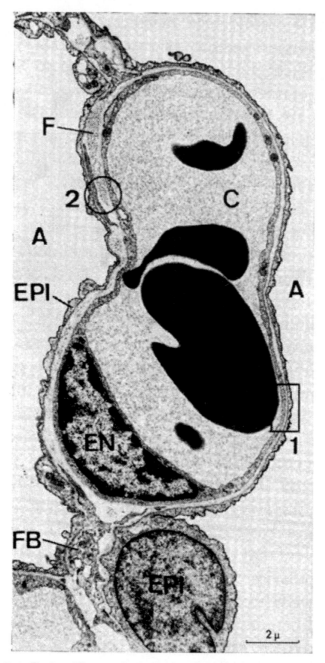

**Figure 5-1. Electron Micrograph of a Portion of an Alveolar Wall.** *(A)* Alveolar space; *(EPI)* type I alveolar epithelial cell nucleus and cytoplasm; *(C)* capillary lumen; *(EN)* endothelial cell nucleus; *(FB)* fibroblast; *(F)* collagen fibrils; *(1)* thin region of blood-gas barrier; *(2)* thick region of blood-gas barrier. (From Weibel ER. Morphological basis of alveolar-capillary gas exchange. *Physiolo Res* 1973;53:419–495.)

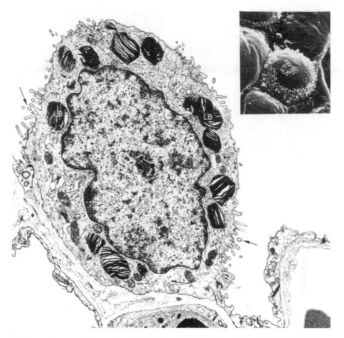

**Figure 5-2. Electron Micrograph of Type 2 Epithelial Cell (10,000×).** Note the lamellated bodies *(LB)*, large nucleus, and microvilli *(arrows)*, which are mainly concentrated around the edge of the cell, and cytoplasm rich in organelles. The inset at top right is a scanning electron micrograph showing the surface view of a type 2 cell with its characteristic distribution of microvilli (3400×). (From Weibel ER, Gil J. Structure–function relationships at the alveolar level. In: West JB, ed. *Bioengineering Aspects of the Lung*, New York, NY: Marcel Dekker, 1977.)

capillary, the interstitium is usually wider and includes fibrils of type I collagen. The thick side is chiefly concerned with fluid exchange across the endothelium, whereas the thin side is responsible for most of the gas exchange (see Figure 6-1).

Interstitial tissue is found elsewhere in the lung, notably in the perivascular and peribronchial spaces around the larger blood vessels and airways and in the interlobular septa. The interstitium of the alveolar wall is continuous with that in the perivascular spaces (see Figure 6-1) and is the route by which fluid drains from the capillaries to the lymphatics.

## Diffuse Interstitial Pulmonary Fibrosis

The nomenclature of this condition is confusing. Synonyms include idiopathic pulmonary fibrosis, interstitial pneumonia, and cryptogenic fibrosing alveolitis. Some physicians reserve the term "fibrosis" for the late stages of the disease. The changes in pulmonary function are described in detail because they are typical of many of the other conditions alluded to later in this chapter.

### Pathology

The principal feature is thickening of the interstitium of the alveolar wall. Initially there is infiltration with lymphocytes and plasma cells. Later, fibroblasts appear and lay down thick collagen bundles (Figure 5-3). These changes may be dispersed irregularly within the lung. In some patients, a cellular exudate consisting of macrophages and other mononuclear cells is

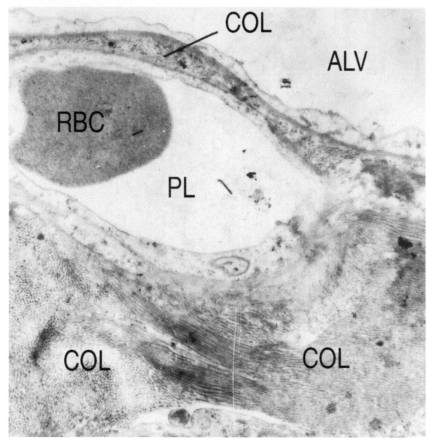

**Figure 5-3. Electron Micrograph from a Patient with Diffuse Interstitial Fibrosis.** Note the thick bundles of collagen. *COL*, collagen; *ALV*, alveolar space; *RBC*, red blood cell; *PL*, plasma. Compare Figure 5-1. (From Gracey DR, Divertie MD, Brown AL Jr. Alveolar–capillary membrane in idiopathic interstitial pulmonary fibrosis. Electron microscopic study of 14 cases. *Am Rev Respir Dis* 1968;98:16–21.)

seen within the alveoli in the early stages of the disease. This is called "desquamation." Eventually, the alveolar architecture is destroyed and the scarring results in multiple air-filled cystic spaces formed by dilated terminal and respiratory bronchioles, so-called honeycomb lung.

## Pathogenesis

This is unknown, although in some cases there is evidence of an immunologic reaction.

## Clinical Features

The disease is not common and tends to affect adults in early or late middle age. The patient often presents with dyspnea with rapid, shallow breathing. The dyspnea typically becomes more significant on exercise (compare Figure 3-3). An irritating, unproductive cough is often present.

On examination, mild cyanosis may be seen at rest in severe cases. It typically worsens on exercise. Fine crepitations are usually heard throughout both lungs, especially toward the end of inspiration. Finger clubbing is common. The chest radiograph (Figure 5-4)

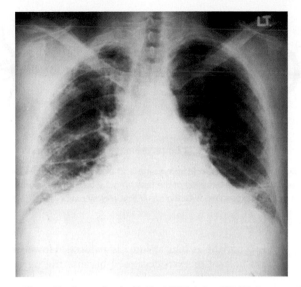

**Figure 5-4.** Chest Radiograph of a Patient With Interstitial Pulmonary Fibrosis. Note the small contracted lung and ribcage and the raised diaphragms. Compare the normal appearance in Figures 4-8A and 4-9A. Opacification of the lung tissue is seen especially at the right base.

shows a reticular or reticulonodular pattern, especially at the bases. Patchy shadows near the diaphragm may be caused by basal collapse. Late in the disease, a honeycomb appearance is often seen; this is caused by multiple airspaces surrounded by thickened tissue. The lungs are typically small, and the diaphragms are raised.

Cor pulmonale or pneumonia may complicate the picture, and the patient may develop respiratory failure terminally. The diseases often progress insidiously, although an acute form does occur.

## Pulmonary Function

### Ventilatory Capacity and Mechanics

Spirometry typically reveals a restrictive pattern (see Figure 1-2). The FVC is markedly reduced, but the gas is exhaled rapidly so that although the $FEV_1$ is low, the FEV/FVC% may exceed the normal value. The almost square shape of the forced expiratory spirogram is in striking contrast to the obstructive pattern (compare Figure 4-16). The $FEF_{25-75\%}$ is normal or high. The flow–volume curve does not show the scooped-out shape of obstructive disease, and the flow rate is often higher than normal when related to absolute lung volume. This is shown in Figure 1-5, where it can be seen that the downslope of the curve for restrictive disease lies above the normal curve.

All lung volumes are reduced, including the TLC, FRC, and RV, but the relative proportions are more or less preserved. The pressure–volume curve of the lung is flattened and displaced downward (see Figure 3-1), so that at any given volume, the transpulmonary pressure is abnormally high. The maximum elastic recoil pressure that can be generated at TLC is typically higher than normal. Airway resistance is normal or low when related to lung volume.

All these results are consistent with the pathologic appearance of fibrosis of the alveolar walls (Figures 2-5 and 5-3). The fibrous tissue reduces the distensibility of the lung just as a scar on the skin reduces its extensibility. As a result, the lung volumes are small, and abnormally large pressures are required to distend the lung. The airways may not be specifically

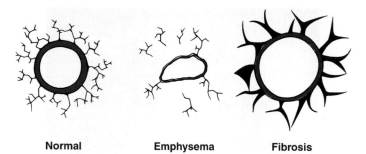

Normal              Emphysema              Fibrosis

**Figure 5-5. Airway Caliber in Emphysema and Interstitial Fibrosis.** In emphysema, the airways tend to collapse because of the loss of radial traction. By contrast, in fibrosis, radial traction may be excessive, with the result that airway caliber is large when related to lung volume.

involved, but they tend to narrow as lung volume is reduced. However, airway resistance at a given lung volume is normal or even decreased because the retractile forces exerted on the airway walls by the surrounding parenchyma are abnormally high (Figure 5-5). The pathologic correlate of this is the honeycomb appearance caused by the dilated terminal and respiratory bronchioles surrounded by thickened scar tissue.

### Gas Exchange

The arterial $P_{O_2}$ and $P_{CO_2}$ are typically reduced, and the pH is normal. The hypoxemia is usually mild at rest until the disease is advanced. However, on exercise, the $P_{O_2}$ often falls dramatically and cyanosis may be evident. In well-established disease, both the physiologic dead space and the physiologic shunt are increased.

The relative contribution of diffusion impairment and ventilation–perfusion ($\dot{V}_A/\dot{Q}$) inequality to the hypoxemia of these patients has long been debated. It is natural to argue that the histologic appearances shown in Figures 2-5 and 5-3 slow the diffusion of oxygen from the alveolar gas to the capillary blood because the thickness of the barrier may be increased many fold (compare Figure 5-1). In addition, the increasing hypoxemia during exercise is consistent with the mechanism of impaired diffusion because exercise reduces the time spent by the red cells in the pulmonary capillary (Figure 2-4).

## Features of Pulmonary Function in Diffuse Interstitial Fibrosis

- Dyspnea with shallow, rapid breathing
- Reductions in all lung volumes
- $FEV_1/FVC$ ratio normal or even increased
- Airway resistance normal or low when related to lung volume
- Reduced lung compliance
- Very negative intrapleural pressure at TLC
- Arterial hypoxemia chiefly due to $\dot{V}_A/\dot{Q}$ inequality
- Diffusion impairment possibly contributing to the hypoxemia during exercise
- Normal or low arterial $P_{CO_2}$
- Reduced diffusing capacity for carbon monoxide
- Increased pulmonary vascular resistance

However, we now know that impaired diffusion is not the chief cause of the hypoxemia in these conditions. First, the normal lung has enormous reserves of diffusion in that the $P_{O_2}$ of the blood nearly reaches that in alveolar gas early in its transit through the capillary (see Figure 2-4). In addition, these patients have substantial inequality of ventilation and blood flow within the lung. How could they not, with the disorganization of architecture shown in Figures 2-5 and 5-3? The inequalities have been demonstrated by single-breath nitrogen washouts and measurements of topographical function with radioactive gases.

To apportion blame for the hypoxemia between the two possible mechanisms, it is necessary to measure the degree of $\dot{V}_A/\dot{Q}$ inequality and determine how much of the hypoxemia is attributable to this. This has been done by using the multiple inert gas elimination technique in a series of patients with interstitial lung disease. Figure 5-6 shows that at rest the hypoxemia could be adequately explained by the degree of $\dot{V}_A/\dot{Q}$ inequality in these patients. However, Figure 5-7 shows that on exercise the observed alveolar $P_{O_2}$ was generally below the value predicted from the measured amount of $\dot{V}_A/\dot{Q}$ inequality, and thus an additional cause of hypoxemia must have been present. Most likely this was diffusion impairment in these patients. However, hypoxemia caused by diffusion impairment was evident only on exercise, and even then it accounted for only about one-third of the alveolar–arterial difference for $P_{O_2}$.

The low arterial $P_{CO_2}$ in these patients (typically in the middle or early 30s) occurs despite the evident $\dot{V}_A/\dot{Q}$ inequality and is caused by increased ventilation to the alveoli (compare Figure 2-9). The cause of the increased ventilation is uncertain. There is some evidence that the control of ventilation is abnormal because of the stimulation of receptors within the lung (see later text). Stimulation of the peripheral chemoreceptors by the arterial hypoxemia may also be a factor. The arterial pH is usually normal at rest but may increase considerably on exercise as a result of the hyperventilation and consequent respiratory alkalosis (compare Figure 3-3), although metabolic acidosis caused by lactic acid accumulation may also occur. In terminal respiratory failure, the pH may fall.

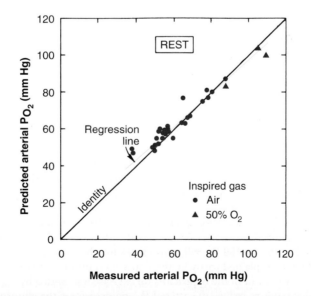

**Figure 5-6. Study of the Mechanism of Hypoxemia in a Series of Patients with Interstitial Lung Disease.** This figure shows that the arterial $P_{O_2}$ predicted from the pattern of $\dot{V}_A/\dot{Q}$ inequality agreed well with the measured arterial $P_{O_2}$. Thus at rest, all of the hypoxemia could be explained by the uneven ventilation and blood flow.

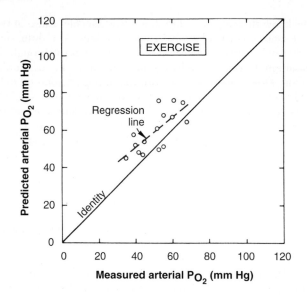

**Figure 5-7. Results Obtained on Exercise in the Same Patients as Shown in Figure 5-5.** Under these conditions the measured arterial $P_{O_2}$ was below that predicted from the pattern of $\dot{V}_A/\dot{Q}$ inequality. This indicates an additional mechanism for hypoxemia, presumably diffusion impairment.

The diffusing capacity for carbon monoxide is often strikingly reduced in these patients to the neighborhood of 5 ml/min per mm Hg (normal value 25–30 depending on age and stature). This may be a useful diagnostic pointer: if the diffusing capacity is not low, the diagnosis should be regarded with suspicion. The reduction is caused in part by the thickening of the blood–gas barrier (Figure 2-5). In addition, the blood volume of the pulmonary capillaries decreases because many of the vessels are obliterated by the fibrotic process. A further factor in the lower measured diffusing capacity is probably the $\dot{V}_A/\dot{Q}$ inequality, which causes uneven emptying of the lung. The diffusing capacity should not be taken to reflect only the properties of the blood–gas barrier.

*Exercise*

Patients with mild diffuse interstitial fibrosis may show much more evidence of impaired pulmonary function on exercise than at rest. The changes shown in Figure 3-3B are typical, although this patient had hypersensitivity pneumonitis (see later text). Note that the maximal $O_2$ intake and $CO_2$ output were severely limited compared with the normal values of Figure 3-3A. The increase in ventilation on exercise was greatly exaggerated. This exaggeration was chiefly caused by the high rate of breathing, which rose to over 60 breaths per minute during maximal exercise.

As a result of the high ventilation, which was out of proportion to the increase in $O_2$ uptake and $CO_2$ output, the alveolar and arterial $P_{CO_2}$ fell and the alveolar $P_{O_2}$ rose. However, as noted earlier, the arterial $P_{O_2}$ fell, thus increasing the alveolar–arterial difference for $P_{O_2}$. This result can be explained partly by the impaired diffusion characteristics of the lung (Figure 5-6). However, most of the hypoxemia on exercise was caused by $\dot{V}_A/\dot{Q}$ inequality.

One factor that tends to reduce the arterial $P_{O_2}$ on exercise is the abnormal small rise in cardiac output. These patients typically have an increased pulmonary vascular resistance. This is particularly evident on exercise, during which the pulmonary artery pressure may rise substantially. The high resistance is caused by the obliteration of much of the pulmonary capillary bed by the interstitial fibrosis (see Figure 2-5). Another factor is hypertrophy of vascular smooth muscle and consequent narrowing of the small arteries. It is important to appreciate that an abnormally low cardiac output in the presence of $\dot{V}_A/\dot{Q}$ inequality can cause hypoxemia. One way of looking at this is that a low cardiac output results in a low $P_{O_2}$ in the mixed venous blood (see Chapter 9). As a consequence, a lung unit with a given $\dot{V}_A/\dot{Q}$ will oxygenate the blood less than when the mixed venous $P_{O_2}$ is normal.

The importance of this factor can be seen if we consider some results obtained in our laboratory in a patient with interstitial lung disease. During exercise that raised the $O_2$ uptake from about 300 to 700 ml/min, the arterial $P_{O_2}$ fell from 50 to 35 mm Hg. The rise in cardiac output was only from 4.6 to 5.7 liters/min; the normal value for this level of exercise is approximately 10 liters/min. As a result, the $P_{O_2}$ in the mixed venous blood fell to 17 mm Hg (normal value is approximately 35 mm Hg). Calculations show that if the cardiac output had increased to 10 liters/min (and the pattern of $\dot{V}_A/\dot{Q}$ inequality remained unchanged), the arterial $P_{O_2}$ would have been some 10 mm Hg higher.

If the diffusing capacity for carbon monoxide is measured in these patients during exercise, it typically remains low, whereas it may double or triple in normal subjects.

### Control of Ventilation

We have already seen that these patients typically have shallow rapid breathing, especially on exercise. The reason for this is not certain, but it is possible that the pattern is caused by reflexes originating in pulmonary irritant receptors or J (juxtacapillary) receptors. The former lie in the bronchi or in the epithelial lining and may be stimulated by the increased traction on the airways caused by the increased elastic recoil of the lung (Figure 5-5). The J receptors are in the alveolar walls and could be stimulated by the fibrotic changes in the interstitium. No direct evidence of increased activity of either receptor is yet available in humans, but work in experimental animals suggests that these reflexes could cause rapid shallow breathing.

The rapid shallow pattern of breathing reduces the respiratory work in patients with reduced lung compliance. However, it also increases ventilation of the anatomic dead space at the expense of the alveoli, so a compromise must be reached.

## Other Types of Parenchymal Restrictive Disease

The changes in pulmonary function in diffuse interstitial pulmonary fibrosis have been dealt with at some length because this disease serves as an example for other forms of parenchymal restrictive disease. These diseases are now considered briefly here, and differences in their pattern of pulmonary function are discussed.

### Sarcoidosis

This disease is characterized by the presence of granulomatous tissue having a characteristic histologic appearance. It often occurs in several organs.

### Pathology

The characteristic lesion is a noncaseating epithelioid granuloma composed of large histiocytes with giant cells and lymphocytes. This lesion may occur in the lymph nodes, lungs, skin, eyes, liver, spleen, and elsewhere. In advanced pulmonary disease, fibrotic changes in the alveolar walls are seen.

### Pathogenesis

This is unknown, although an immunologic basis appears likely. One possibility is that an unknown antigen is recognized by an alveolar macrophage, and this results in the activation of a T lymphocyte and the production of interleukin-2. The activated macrophage may also release various products that stimulate fibroblasts, thus explaining the deposition of fibrous tissue in the interstitium.

## Clinical Features

Four stages of sarcoidosis can be identified.

- *Stage 0:* These patients have no obvious intrathoracic involvement, although a CT scan may show enlarged mediastinal lymph nodes (lymphadenopathy).

- *Stage 1:* There is bilateral hilar adenopathy often with right paratracheal adenopathy. This is often accompanied by erythema nodosum of the legs. Arthritis, uveitis, and parotic gland enlargement may also occur. There are no disturbances of pulmonary function.

- *Stage 2:* The pulmonary parenchyma is also involved, the most common radiologic appearance being widespread mottled shadows, most significant in the mid and upper zones. Symptoms include breathlessness and a dry, unproductive cough.

- *Stage 3:* Here there are pulmonary infiltrates without adenopathy. Fibrosis is seen predominantly in the upper lobes, and cavities or bullae may be present.

## Pulmonary Function

There is no impairment of function in stages 0 and 1 of the disease. In stages 2 and 3, typical changes of the restrictive type are seen, although the radiographic appearance sometimes suggests more interference with function than actually exists.

Ultimately, significant pulmonary fibrosis may develop, with a severe restrictive pattern of function. All lung volumes are small, but the FEV/FVC% is preserved. Lung compliance is strikingly reduced, the pressure–volume curve being flattened and shifted downward and to the right (see Figure 3-1). The resting arterial $P_{O_2}$ is low and often falls considerably on exercise. The arterial $P_{CO_2}$ is normal or low, although, terminally, it may rise as respiratory failure supervenes. The diffusing capacity for carbon monoxide (transfer factor) is reduced significantly. Cor pulmonale may develop in advanced disease.

## Hypersensitivity Pneumonitis

This is also known as extrinsic allergic alveolitis. It is a hypersensitivity reaction affecting the lung parenchyma that occurs in response to inhaled organic dusts. A good example is farmer's lung. The exposure is usually occupational and heavy. The disease is an example of type 3 hypersensitivity (or combination of types 3 and 4), and precipitins can be demonstrated in the serum.

The term "extrinsic" implies that the etiologic agent is external and can be identified, in contrast to "intrinsic" fibrosing alveolitis (diffuse interstitial fibrosis discussed above), where the cause is unknown. Farmer's lung is due to the spores of thermophilic *Actinomyces* in moldy hay. Bird breeder's lung is caused by avian antigens from feathers and excreta. Air conditioner's lung and bagassosis (in sugarcane workers) are also recognized.

## Pathology

The alveolar walls are thickened and infiltrated with lymphocytes, plasma cells, and occasional eosinophils together with collections of histiocytes that, in some areas, form small granulomas. The small bronchioles are usually affected, and there may be exudate in the lumen. Fibrotic changes occur in advanced cases.

## Clinical Features

The disease occurs in either acute or chronic forms. In the former, symptoms of dyspnea, fever, shivering, and cough appear 4 to 6 hours after exposure and continue for 24 to 48 hours. The patient is frequently dyspneic at rest, with fine crepitations throughout both lung fields. The disease may also occur in a chronic form without prior acute attacks. These patients present with progressive dyspnea, usually over a period of years. In the acute form, the chest radiograph may be normal, but frequently a military nodular infiltrate is present. In the chronic form, fibrosis of the upper lobes is common.

### Pulmonary Function

In well-developed disease, the typical restrictive pattern is seen. This includes reduced lung volumes, low compliance, hypoxemia that worsens on exercise, normal or low arterial $P_{CO_2}$, and a reduced diffusing capacity (Figure 3-3). In the early stages, variable degrees of airway obstruction may be present.

### Interstitial Disease Caused by Drugs, Poisons, and Radiation

Various drugs may cause an acute pulmonary reaction, which can proceed to interstitial fibrosis. These drugs include busulfan (used in the treatment of chronic myeloid leukemia), the antibiotic nitrofurantoin, the cardiac antiarrhythmic agent amiodarone, and the cytostatic drug bleomycin. Other antineoplastic drugs can also cause fibrosis. Oxygen in high concentrations causes acute toxic changes with subsequent interstitial fibrosis (see Figure 5-3). Ingestion of the weedkiller paraquat results in the rapid development of lethal interstitial fibrosis. Therapeutic radiation causes acute pneumonitis followed by fibrosis if lung is included in the field.

### Collagen Diseases

Interstitial fibrosis with a typical restrictive pattern may be found in patients with systemic sclerosis (generalized scleroderma). Dyspnea is often severe and out of proportion to the changes in radiologic appearance or lung function. Other connective tissue diseases that may produce fibrosis include systemic lupus erythematosus and rheumatoid arthritis.

### Lymphangitis Carcinomatosa

This refers to the spread of carcinoma tissue through pulmonary lymphatics and may complicate carcinomas, chiefly of the stomach or breast. Dyspnea is prominent, and the typical restrictive pattern of lung function may be seen.

## ▶ Diseases of the Pleura

## Pneumothorax

Air can enter the pleural space either from the lung or, less commonly, through the chest wall as a result of a penetrating wound. The pressure in the intrapleural space is normally subatmospheric as a result of the elastic recoil forces of the lung and chest wall. When air enters the space, the lung collapses and the rib cage springs out. (See *Respiratory Physiology: The Essentials*, 9th ed., p. 111). These changes are evident on a chest radiograph (Figure 5-8), which shows partial or complete collapse of the lung, overexpansion of the rib cage and depression of the diaphragm on the affected side, and sometimes displacement of the mediastinum away from the pneumothorax. An example is shown in Figure 5-8. These changes are most evident if the pneumothorax is large, particularly if a tension pneumothorax is present (see later text).

### Spontaneous Pneumothorax

This most common form of pneumothorax is caused by the rupture of a small bleb on the surface of the lung near the apex. It typically occurs in tall young males and may be related to the high mechanical stresses that occur in the upper zone of the upright lung

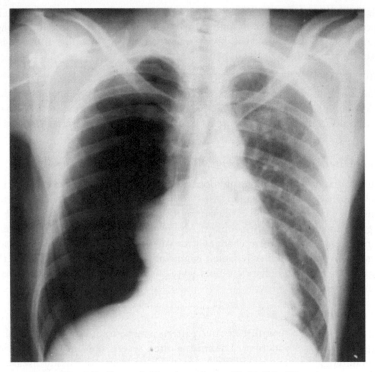

**Figure 5-8. Chest Radiograph Showing a Large Right-Sided Spontaneous Pneumothorax.** Note the small, collapsed right lung, depression of the right hemidiaphragm, and overexpansion of the rib cage on the right.

(see Figure 3-4). The presenting symptom is often sudden pain on one side accompanied by dyspnea. On auscultation, breath sounds are reduced on the affected side and the diagnosis is readily confirmed by a radiograph.

The pneumothorax gradually absorbs because the sum of the partial pressures in the venous blood is considerably less than atmospheric pressure. Recurrent attacks may need surgical treatment to promote adhesions between the two pleural surfaces (pleurodesis).

## Spontaneous Pneumothorax

- Typically occurs in young people in their 20s
- Accompanied by dyspnea and pain
- Gradually absorbed by the blood
- Recurrent attacks may require surgery
- Tension pneumothorax is a medical emergency

### *Tension Pneumothorax*

In a small proportion of spontaneous pneumothoraces, the communication between the lung and the pleural space functions as a check valve. As a consequence, air enters the space during inspiration but cannot escape during expiration. The result is a large pneumothorax in which the pressure may considerably exceed atmospheric pressure and thus interfere with venous return to the thorax.

This medical emergency is recognized by increasing respiratory distress, tachycardia, and signs of mediastinal shift, such as tracheal deviation and displacement of the apex beat. The radiograph is usually diagnostic. Treatment consists of relieving the pressure by inserting a tube through the chest wall. This tube is connected to an underwater seal that allows air to escape from the chest but not to enter it.

### Pneumothorax Complicating Lung Disease

This occurs in a variety of conditions, including rupture of a bulla in COPD or a cyst in advanced fibrotic disease. It also sometimes occurs during mechanical ventilation with high airway pressures (see Chapter 10).

### Pulmonary Function

As would be expected, a pneumothorax reduces the $FEV_1$ and FVC. In practice, pulmonary function tests are rarely helpful in treating these patients because the radiograph is so informative.

## Pleural Effusion

This refers to fluid rather than air in the pleural space. It is not a disease in its own right, but it frequently accompanies serious disease, and an explanation should always be sought.

The patient often reports dyspnea if the effusion is large, and there may be pleuritic pain from the underlying disease. The chest signs are often informative and include reduced movement of the chest on the affected side, absence of breath sounds, and dullness to percussion. The radiograph is diagnostic.

Pleural effusions can be divided into exudates and transudates according to whether their protein content is high or low. In addition, the lactic dehydrogenase concentration tends to be higher in transudates. Exudates typically occur with malignancies and infections, whereas transudates complicate severe heart failure and other edematous states. It is often necessary to aspirate an effusion, but treatment should be directed at the underlying cause. Pulmonary function is impaired as in pneumothorax, but the measurements are not required in practice.

Variants of pleural effusion include empyema (pyothorax), hemothorax, and chylothorax, which refer to the presence of pus, blood, and lymph, respectively, in the pleural space.

## Pleural Thickening

Occasionally, a long-standing pleural effusion results in a rigid, contracted fibrotic pleura that splints the lung and prevents its expansion. This can result in a severe restrictive type of functional impairment, particularly if the disease is bilateral. Surgical stripping may be necessary.

## ▶ Diseases of the Chest Wall

## Scoliosis

Bony deformity of the chest can cause restrictive disease. "Scoliosis" refers to lateral curvature of the spine and kyphosis to posterior curvature. Scoliosis is more serious, especially if the angulation is high in the vertebral column. It is frequently associated with a backward protuberance of the ribs, giving the appearance of an added kyphosis. In most cases, the cause is unknown, although the condition is occasionally caused by bony tuberculosis or neuromuscular disease.

The patient initially reports dyspnea on exertion; breathing tends to be rapid and shallow. Hypoxemia later develops, and eventually carbon dioxide retention and cor pulmonale may supervene. Bronchitis is common if the patient smokes.

Pulmonary function tests typically show a reduction in all lung volumes. Airway resistance is nearly normal if related to lung volume. However, there is inequality of ventilation, partly because of airway closure in dependent regions. Parts of the lung are compressed and there are often areas of atelectasis.

The hypoxemia is caused by ventilation–perfusion inequality. In advanced disease, a reduced ventilatory response to $CO_2$ can often be demonstrated. This reduction reflects the increased work of breathing caused by deformity of the chest wall. Not only is the chest wall stiff, but also the respiratory muscles operate inefficiently. The pulmonary vascular bed is restricted, causing a rise in pulmonary artery pressure, which is exaggerated by the alveolar hypoxia. Venous congestion and peripheral edema may develop. The patient may succumb to an intercurrent pulmonary infection or respiratory failure.

## Ankylosing Spondylitis

In this disease of unknown etiology, there is a gradual but relentless onset of immobility of the vertebral joints and fixation of the ribs. As a result, the movement of the chest wall is grossly reduced. There is a reduction of FVC and TLC, but the FEV/FVC% and the airway resistance are normal. The compliance of the chest wall may fall, and there is often some uneven ventilation, probably secondary to the reduced lung volume. The lung itself remains normal in nearly all cases, and diaphragmatic movement is preserved. Respiratory failure does not occur.

## ▶ Neuromuscular Disorders

Diseases affecting the muscles of respiration or their nerve supply include poliomyelitis, Guillain-Barré syndrome, amyotrophic lateral sclerosis, myasthenia gravis, and muscular dystrophies (see Table 2-1 and Figure 2-3). All these diseases can lead to dyspnea and respiratory failure. The inability of the patient to take in a deep breath is reflected in a reduced FVC, TLC, inspiratory capacity, and $FEV_1$.

It should be remembered that the most important muscle of respiration is the diaphragm, and patients with progressive disease often do not report dyspnea until the diaphragm is involved. By then their ventilatory reserve may be severely compromised. The progress of the disease can be monitored by measuring the FVC and the blood gases. The maximal inspiratory and expiratory pressures that the patient can develop are also reduced. Assisted ventilation (see Chapter 10) may become necessary.

## KEY CONCEPTS

1. Diffuse interstitial pulmonary fibrosis is an example of restrictive lung disease characterized by dyspnea, reduced exercise tolerance, small lungs, and reduced lung compliance.

2. The alveolar walls show marked infiltration with collagen and obliteration of capillaries.

3. Airway resistance is not increased; indeed, a forced expiration can result in abnormally high flow rates because of the increased radial traction on the airway.

4. Diffusion of oxygen across the blood–gas barrier is impeded by the thickening and may result in hypoxemia, especially on exercise. However, ventilation–perfusion inequality is the major factor in the impaired gas exchange.

5. Other restrictive disorders are caused by diseases of the pleura or chest wall or neuromuscular disease.

## QUESTIONS

1. The type II alveolar epithelial cell:

   A. Provides most of the structural support for the normal alveolar wall.
   B. Cannot multiply.
   C. Is formed when a type I epithelial cell is damaged.
   D. Secretes surfactant.
   E. Is metabolically inactive.

2. Histologic changes in diffuse interstitial pulmonary fibrosis typically include:

   A. Infiltration of the alveolar wall with lymphocytes and plasma cells.
   B. Breakdown of many alveolar walls.
   C. Mucous gland hypertrophy in the bronchi.
   D. Mucous plugging of airways.
   E. Increased volume of the pulmonary capillary bed.

3. Features of diffuse interstitial pulmonary fibrosis include:

   A. Cough productive of copious sputum.
   B. Hemoptysis.
   C. Rhonchi in both lungs.
   D. Dyspnea especially on exercise.
   E. Depressed diaphragms on the radiograph.

4. Pulmonary function tests in diffuse interstitial pulmonary fibrosis typically show:

   A. Increased $FEV_1$.
   B. Increased FVC.
   C. Increased $FEV_1/FVC\%$.
   D. Increased TLC.
   E. Increased airway resistance when related to lung volume.

5. The arterial hypoxemia of a patient with diffuse interstitial pulmonary fibrosis:

   A. Typically worsens on exercise.
   B. Is chiefly caused by diffusion impairment.
   C. Is associated with a large increase in diffusing capacity during exercise.
   D. Is usually associated with carbon dioxide retention.
   E. Is improved during exercise because of the abnormally large increase in cardiac output.

6. In a patient with diffuse interstitial fibrosis of the lung, the maximal expiratory flow rate at a given lung volume may be higher than in a normal subject because:

   A. Expiratory muscles have a large mechanical advantage.
   B. Airways have a small diameter.
   C. Dynamic compression of the airways is more likely than in a normal subject.
   D. Radial traction on the airways is increased.
   E. Airway resistance is increased.

7. The diffusing capacity for carbon monoxide in a patient with diffuse interstitial lung disease:

   A. Is typically substantially increased.
   B. Shows an abnormally large increase during exercise.
   C. Is unaffected by thickening of the blood–gas barrier.
   D. Is reduced in part because of obliteration of pulmonary capillaries.
   E. Falls only late in the disease.

**8.** Features of pneumothorax include:

    A. It reduces the volume of the chest wall on the affected side.

    B. It causes an increased blood flow in the affected lung.

    C. When present in the tension form, it is a medical emergency.

    D. Spontaneous pneumothorax is mainly seen in older women.

    E. The FVC is increased.

# Vascular Diseases

**6**

The pathophysiology of the pulmonary vasculature is of great importance. Pulmonary edema is not a disease in its own right, but it complicates many heart and lung diseases and can be life-threatening. Pulmonary embolism is frequently underdiagnosed and may be fatal. The pathophysiology of primary pulmonary hypertension is poorly understood, and much research is being directed at drug therapy.

> ## Pulmonary Edema

*Pulmonary edema is an abnormal accumulation of fluid in the extravascular spaces and tissues of the lung. It is an important complication of a variety of heart and lung diseases and may be life-threatening.*

## Pathophysiology

Figure 5-1 reminds us that the pulmonary capillary is lined by endothelial cells and surrounded by an interstitial space. As the figure shows, the interstitium is narrow on one side of the capillary, where it is formed by the fusion of the two basement membranes, while on the other side it is wider and contains type I collagen fibers. This latter region is particularly important for fluid exchange. Between the interstitial and alveolar spaces are the alveolar epithelium, composed predominantly of type 1 cells, and the superficial layer of surfactant (not shown in Figure 5-1).

The capillary endothelium is highly permeable to water and many solutes, including small molecules and ions. Proteins have a restricted movement across the endothelium. By contrast, the alveolar epithelium is much less permeable, and even small ions are largely prevented from crossing by passive diffusion. In addition, the epithelium actively pumps water from the alveolar to interstitial space using a sodium, potassium, ATPase pump.

Hydrostatic forces tend to move fluid out of the capillary into the interstitial space, and osmotic forces tend to keep it in. The movement of fluid across the endothelium is governed by the Starling equation:

$$\dot{Q} = K[(P_c - P_i) - \sigma(\pi_c - \pi_i)],$$

(Eq. 6.1)

where $\dot{Q}$ is the net flow out of the capillary; K the filtration coefficient; $P_c$ and $P_i$ the hydrostatic pressures in the capillary and interstitial space, respectively; $\pi_c$ and $\pi_i$ the corresponding colloid osmotic pressures; and $\sigma$ the reflection coefficient. This last variable indicates the effectiveness of the membrane in preventing (reflecting) the passage of proteins compared with that of water across the endothelium, and the coefficient is reduced in diseases that damage the cells and increase the permeability.

Although this equation is valuable conceptually, its practical use is limited. Of the four pressures, only one, the colloid osmotic pressure within the capillary, is known with any certainty. Its value is 25 to 28 mm Hg. The capillary hydrostatic pressure is probably halfway between arterial and venous pressures but varies markedly from top to bottom of the upright lung. The colloid osmotic pressure of the interstitial fluid is not known but is approximately 20 mm Hg in lung lymph. However, there is some question as to whether this lymph has the same protein concentration as the interstitial fluid around the capillaries. The interstitial hydrostatic pressure is unknown but is thought by some physiologists to be substantially below atmospheric pressure. The value of $\sigma$ in the pulmonary capillaries is approximately 0.7. It is probable that the net pressure from the Starling equilibrium is outward, causing a lymph flow of perhaps 20 ml/hr.

The fluid that leaves the capillaries moves within the interstitial space of the alveolar wall and tracks to the perivascular and peribronchial interstitium (Figure 6-1). This tissue normally forms a thin sheath around the pulmonary arteries, veins, and bronchi and contains the lymphatics. The alveoli themselves are devoid of lymphatics, but once the fluid reaches the perivascular and peribronchial interstitium, some of it is carried in the lymphatics while some moves through the loose interstitial tissue. The lymphatics actively pump the lymph toward the bronchial and hilar lymph nodes.

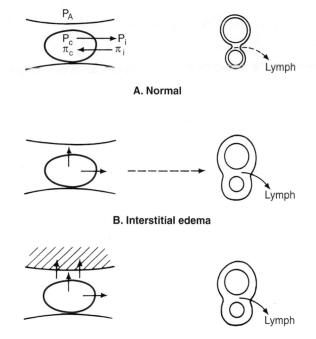

**A. Normal**

**B. Interstitial edema**

**C. Alveolar edema**

**Figure 6-1. Stages of Pulmonary Edema. A.** There is normally a small lymph flow from the lung.
**B.** Interstitial edema. Here there is an increased flow with engorgement of the perivascular and peribronchial spaces and some widening of the alveolar wall interstitium. **C.** Some fluid crosses the epithelium, producing alveolar edema.

If excessive amounts of fluid leak from the capillaries, two factors tend to limit this flow. The first is a fall in the colloid osmotic pressure of the interstitial fluid as the protein is diluted as a result of the faster filtration of water compared with protein. However, this factor does not operate if the permeability of the capillary is greatly increased. The second is a rise in hydrostatic pressure in the interstitial space, which reduces the net filtration pressure. Both factors act to reduce fluid movement out of the capillaries.

Two stages in the formation of pulmonary edema are recognized (Figure 6-1). The first is *interstitial edema*, which is characterized by the engorgement of the perivascular and peribronchial interstitial tissue (cuffing), as shown in Figure 6-2. Widened lymphatics can be seen, and lymph flow increases. In addition, some widening of the interstitium of the thick side of the capillary occurs. Pulmonary function is little affected at this stage, and the condition is difficult to recognize, although some radiologic changes may be seen (see later text).

The second stage is *alveolar edema* (Figure 6-3). Here fluid moves across the epithelium into the alveoli, which are filled one by one. As a result of surface tension forces, the edematous alveoli shrink. Ventilation is prevented, and to the extent that the alveoli remain perfused, shunting of blood occurs and hypoxemia is inevitable. The edema fluid may move into the small and large airways and be coughed up as voluminous frothy sputum. The sputum is often pink because of the presence of red blood cells. What prompts the transition from interstitial to alveolar edema is not fully understood, but it may be that

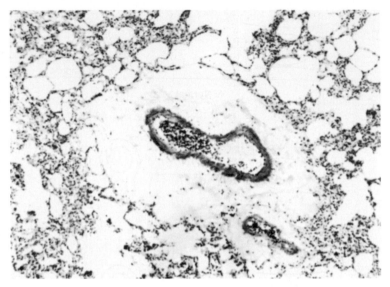

**Figure 6-2. Example of Engorgement of the Perivascular Space of a Small Pulmonary Blood Vessel by Interstitial Edema.** Some alveolar edema is also present.

the lymphatics become overloaded and that the pressure in the interstitial space increases so much that fluid spills over into the alveoli. Probably the alveolar epithelium is damaged and its permeability is increased. This would explain the presence of protein and red cells in the alveolar fluid.

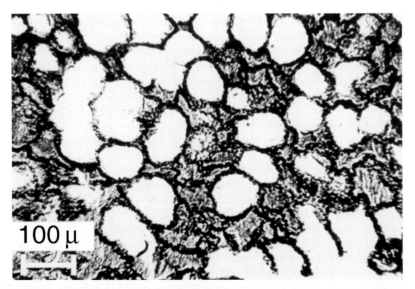

**Figure 6-3. Section of Dog Lung Showing Alveolar Edema.** Note that some alveoli are filled completely and others are spared. The edematous alveoli tend to be smaller. (From Staub NC. The pathophysiology of pulmonary edema. *Hum Pathol* 1970;1:419–432.)

## States of Pulmonary Edema

1. Interstitial edema

   Increased lymph flow from the lung

   Perivascular and peribronchial cuffing

   Septal lines on the chest radiograph

   Little effect on pulmonary function

2. Alveolar edema

   Often severe dyspnea and orthopnea

   Patient may cough up pink, frothy fluid

   Marked opacification on the radiograph

   Often severe hypoxemia

## Pathogenesis

This is best discussed under six headings, as shown in Table 6-1.

### Increased Capillary Hydrostatic Pressure

This is the most common cause of pulmonary edema and frequently complicates heart disease, such as acute myocardial infarction, hypertensive left ventricular failure, and mitral valve disease. In all these conditions, left atrial pressure rises, causing an increase in pulmonary venous and capillary pressures. This can be recognized at cardiac catheterization by measuring the wedge pressure (the pressure in a catheter that has been wedged in a small pulmonary artery), which is approximately equal to pulmonary venous pressure.

Whether pulmonary edema occurs in these conditions depends on the rate of rise of the pressure. For example, in patients with mitral stenosis in whom the venous pressure is gradually raised over a period of years, remarkably high values may occur without clinical evidence of edema. This is partly because the caliber or number of the lymphatics increases to accommodate the higher lymph flow. However, these patients often have marked interstitial edema. By contrast, a patient with an acute myocardial infarction may develop alveolar edema with a smaller but more sudden rise in pulmonary venous pressure.

| Table 6.1 | Causes of Pulmonary Edema |
|---|---|
| **Mechanism** | **Precipitating Event** |
| Increased capillary hydrostatic pressure | Myocardial infarction, mitral stenosis, fluid overload, pulmonary venoocclusive disease |
| Increased capillary permeability | Inhaled or circulating toxins, sepsis, radiation, oxygen toxicity, ARDS |
| Reduced lymph drainage | Increased central venous pressure, lymphangitis carcinomatosa |
| Decreased interstitial pressure | Rapid removal of pleural effusion or pneumothorax, hyperinflation |
| Decreased colloid osmotic pressure | Overtransfusion hypoalbuminemia |
| Uncertain etiology | High altitude, neurogenic, overinflation, heroin |

Noncardiogenic causes also occur. Edema may be precipitated by excessive intravenous infusions of saline, plasma, or blood, leading to a rise in capillary pressure. Diseases of the pulmonary veins, such as pulmonary venoocclusive diseases, may also result in edema.

The cause of the edema in all these conditions is partly the increase in hydrostatic pressure, which disturbs the Starling equilibrium. However, when the capillary pressure is raised to high levels, ultrastructural changes occur in the capillary walls, including disruption of the capillary endothelium, alveolar epithelium, or sometimes all layers of the wall. The result is an increase in permeability with movement of fluid, protein, and cells into the alveolar spaces. The condition is known as capillary stress failure.

With moderate rises in capillary pressure and consequent disturbance of the Starling equilibrium, the alveolar edema fluid has a low protein concentration because the permeability characteristics of the capillary wall are largely preserved. This is sometimes known as low-permeability edema. Traditionally, this has been contrasted with the alveolar edema that occurs when the capillary permeability has been increased, as discussed in the next section. In this case, large amounts of protein are lost from the capillaries, and therefore, the alveolar fluid has a relatively high protein concentration (high-permeability edema). The edema fluid also typically contains red blood cells, which escape through the damaged capillary walls. However, it is now clear that a sufficiently large increase in capillary pressure can also result in a high-permeability type of edema because of damage to the capillary walls caused by the high pressure, that is, stress failure. In fact, there is a continuous spectrum from low-permeability to high-permeability edema depending on the degree of increase in the pulmonary capillary pressure.

### Increased Capillary Permeability

Apart from the situation referred to above, an increased capillary permeability also occurs in a variety of conditions. Toxins that are inhaled (such as chlorine, sulfur dioxide, and nitrogen oxides) or that circulate (such as alloxan and endotoxin) cause pulmonary edema in this way. Therapeutic radiation to the lung may cause edema and, ultimately, interstitial fibrosis. Oxygen poisoning produces a similar picture. Another cause is the adult respiratory distress syndrome (ARDS) (see Chapter 8). As discussed, the edema fluid typically has a high protein concentration and contains many blood cells.

### Reduced Lymph Drainage

This can be an exaggerating factor if another cause is present. One of these is an increased central venous pressure, which may occur in ARDS, heart failure, and overtransfusion. This apparently interferes with the normal drainage of the thoracic duct. Another cause is obstruction of lymphatics, as in lymphangitis carcinomatosa.

### Decreased Interstitial Pressure

This would be expected to promote edema from the Starling equation, although whether this occurs in practice is uncertain. However, if patients have a large unilateral pleural effusion or pneumothorax and then the lung is rapidly expanded, sometimes pulmonary edema develops on that side. This may be partly related to the large mechanical forces acting on the interstitial space as the lung is expanded. However, the edema fluid is of the high-permeability type, and it is probable that the high mechanical stresses in the alveolar walls cause ultrastructural changes in the capillary walls (stress failure).

### Decreased Colloid Osmotic Pressure

This is rarely responsible for pulmonary edema on its own, but it can exaggerate the edema that occurs when some other precipitating factor is present. Overtransfusion with saline is an important example. Another example is the hypoproteinemia of the nephrotic syndrome.

## *Uncertain Etiology*

This includes several forms of pulmonary edema. High-altitude pulmonary edema occasionally affects climbers and skiers (Figure 6-4). The wedge pressure is normal, so a raised pulmonary venous pressure is not the culprit. However, the pulmonary artery pressure is high because of hypoxic vasoconstriction. Current evidence shows that the arteriolar constriction is uneven and that regions of the capillary bed that are therefore not protected from the high pressure develop the ultrastructural changes of stress failure. This hypothesis would explain the high protein concentration in the alveolar fluid. Treatment is by descent to a lower altitude. Oxygen should be given if it is available.

Neurogenic pulmonary edema is seen after injuries to the central nervous system, for example, head trauma. Again, the mechanism is probably stress failure of pulmonary capillaries because there is a large rise in capillary pressure associated with heightened activity of the sympathetic nervous system.

Overinflation of the lung can cause pulmonary edema. This is sometimes seen in the intensive care unit when high levels of positive end-expiratory pressure (PEEP) are used (see Chapter 10). Again, the resulting large mechanical forces in the alveolar walls apparently damage the capillary walls.

Heroin overdose can cause pulmonary edema. This condition is particularly seen in addicts who inject the drug intravenously when it is mixed with various diluents. These diluents might be partly responsible; however, edema can also follow oral ingestion.

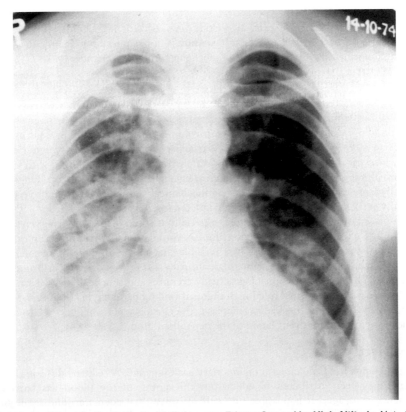

**Figure 6-4. Radiograph of a Patient with Pulmonary Edema Caused by High Altitude.** Note the blotchy shadowing, especially on the right side.

## Clinical Features

These features depend to some extent on the etiology of the edema, but some generalizations can be made. Dyspnea is usually a prominent symptom; breathing is typically rapid and shallow. Mild edema may cause few symptoms at rest, but exertional dyspnea is inevitable. Orthopnea (increased dyspnea while recumbent) is common. Paroxysmal nocturnal dyspnea (the patient awakes at night with severe dyspnea and wheezing) and periodic breathing may occur. Cough is frequent and dry in the early stages. However, in fulminant edema, the patient may cough up large quantities of pink foamy sputum. Cyanosis may be present.

On auscultation, fine crepitations on inspiration are heard at the lung bases in early edema. In more severe cases, musical rhonchi may also be heard. Abnormal heart sounds or murmurs are often present in cardiogenic edema.

Depending on the cause of the edema, the chest radiograph may show an enlarged heart and prominent pulmonary vessels. Interstitial edema causes septal lines to appear on the radiograph. These are short, linear, horizontal markings originating near the pleural surface in the lower zones that are caused by edematous interlobular septa. In more severe edema, blotchy shadowing occurs (Figure 6-4). Sometimes, this shadow radiates from the hilar regions, giving a so-called bat's-wing or butterfly appearance. The explanation of this distribution is not clear but may be related to the perivascular and peribronchial cuffing that is particularly noticeable around the large vessels in the hilar region (Figures 6-1 and 6-2).

## Pulmonary Function

Extensive pulmonary function tests are seldom carried out on patients with pulmonary edema because they are so sick and the information is not required for treatment. The most important abnormalities are in the areas of mechanics and gas exchange.

### Mechanics

Pulmonary edema reduces the distensibility of the lung and moves the pressure–volume curve downward and to the right (compare Figure 3-1). An important factor in this is the alveolar flooding, which causes a reduction in volume of the affected lung units as a result of surface tension forces and reduces their participation in the pressure–volume curve. In addition, interstitial edema per se probably stiffens the lung by interfering with its elastic properties, although it is difficult to obtain clear evidence on this. Edematous lungs require abnormally large expanding pressures during mechanical ventilation and tend to collapse to abnormally small volumes when not actively inflated (see Chapter 10).

Airway resistance is typically increased, especially if some of the larger airways contain edema fluid. Reflex bronchoconstriction due to stimulation of irritant receptors in the bronchial walls may also play a role. It is possible that in the absence of alveolar edema, interstitial edema increases the resistance of small airways as a result of their peribronchial cuff (Figure 6-1). This can be thought of as actually compressing the small airways or, at least, isolating them from the normal traction of the surrounding parenchyma (Figure 6-5). There is some evidence that this mechanism increases the closing volume (Figure 1-10) and thus predisposes to intermittent ventilation of the dependent lung.

### Gas Exchange

Interstitial edema has little effect on pulmonary gas exchange. A reduced diffusing capacity has sometimes been attributed to edematous thickening of the blood–gas barrier, but the evidence is meager. It is possible that cuffs of interstitial edema around small airways (Figures 6-1 and 6-5) can cause intermittent ventilation of dependent regions of the lung, leading to hypoxemia, but the importance of this in practice is uncertain.

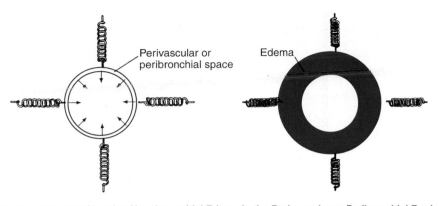

**Figure 6-5. Diagram Showing How Interstitial Edema in the Perivascular or Peribronchial Region Can Reduce the Caliber of the Vessel or Airway.** The cuff isolates the structure from the traction of the surrounding parenchyma.

Alveolar edema causes severe hypoxemia chiefly because of blood flow to unventilated units (see Figure 10-2). These may be edema-filled alveoli or units supplied by airways that are completely obstructed by fluid. Hypoxic vasoconstriction tends to reduce the true shunt, but often this is large, as much as 50% or more of the pulmonary blood flow in severe edema. Mechanical ventilation with PEEP often substantially reduces the amount of shunt chiefly by clearing edema fluid from some of the larger airways (see Figure 10-2), although it may not reduce total lung water.

Lung units with low ventilation–perfusion ratios also contribute to the hypoxemia. These presumably either lie behind airways that are partly obstructed by edema fluid or are units in which the ventilation is reduced by their proximity to edematous alveoli. Such lung units are particularly liable to collapse during treatment with oxygen-enriched mixtures (see Figures 9-4 and 9-5), but oxygen therapy is often essential to relieve the hypoxemia. A factor that often aggravates the hypoxemia caused by edema after acute myocardial infarction is a low cardiac output, which reduces the $P_{O_2}$ in mixed venous blood.

The alveolar $P_{CO_2}$ is often normal or low in pulmonary edema because of increased ventilation to the nonedematous alveoli. This is provoked in part by the arterial hypoxemia and also possibly by stimulation of lung receptors (see next section). However, in fulminating pulmonary edema, carbon dioxide retention and respiratory acidosis may develop.

## Control of Ventilation

Patients with pulmonary edema typically have rapid, shallow breathing. This may be caused by stimulation of J receptors in the alveolar walls and perhaps other vagal afferents. The rapid breathing pattern minimizes the abnormally high elastic work of breathing. Arterial hypoxemia is an additional stimulus to breathing.

## Pulmonary Circulation

Pulmonary vascular resistance rises, and hypoxic vasoconstriction of poorly ventilated or nonventilated areas is one mechanism for this. In addition, perivascular cuffing probably increases the resistance of the extra-alveolar vessels (Figures 6-2 and 6-5). Other possible factors are the partial collapse of edematous alveoli and alveolar wall edema that may compress or distort capillaries.

The topographical distribution of blood flow is sometimes altered by interstitial edema. The normal apex-to-base gradient becomes inverted, with the result that apical flow exceeds basal (Figure 6-6). This is most commonly seen in patients with mitral stenosis. The cause is

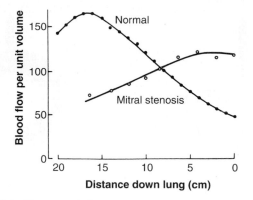

**Figure 6-6. Inversion of the Topographic Distribution of Blood Flow in a Patient with Mitral Stenosis.** The cause is not certain, but interstitial cuffs of edema around the lower zone vessels (Figures 6-2 and 6-5) may be partly responsible.

not fully understood, but it is possible that perivascular cuffs particularly increase the resistance of the lower zone vessels because the lung is less well expanded there (see Figure 3-5). This inverted distribution is not seen in noncardiogenic forms of edema, for example, ARDS.

## ▶ Pulmonary Embolism

This important condition is often preventable and potentially fatal. Small emboli are common and are frequently undiagnosed.

### Pathogenesis

Most pulmonary emboli arise as detached portions of venous thrombi that have formed in the deep veins of the lower extremities. Other sites include the right side of the heart and the pelvic area. Nonthrombotic emboli, such as fat, air, and amniotic fluid, also occur but are relatively uncommon.

Factors that favor the formation of venous thrombi are:

**1.** Stasis of blood

**2.** Alterations in the blood coagulation system

**3.** Abnormalities of the vessel wall

*Stasis of blood* is promoted by immobilization following a fracture or an operation, local pressure, or venous obstruction. It is common in congestive heart failure, shock, hypovolemia, dehydration, and varicose veins. An enlarged fibrillating right atrium often contains some thrombi.

The intravascular *coagulability of blood* is increased in several conditions, such as polycythemia vera and sickle cell disease. The viscosity of the blood increases, thus favoring sluggish flow next to the vessel wall. In other conditions, the mechanism of increased coagulability is poorly understood. Such conditions include malignant diseases, pregnancy, recent trauma, and the use of oral contraceptives. There is no reliable test of an increased tendency for intravascular coagulation.

The *vessel wall may be damaged* by local trauma or by inflammation. Where there is marked local phlebitis with tenderness, redness, warmth, and swelling, the clot may be more securely adherent to the wall.

The presence of thrombosis in the deep veins of the legs or pelvis is often unsuspected until embolism occurs. Sometimes there is swelling of the limb or local tenderness, and there may be signs of inflammation. Acute dorsiflexion of the ankle may elicit calf pain. Ancillary tests, such as venography, the local uptake of radioactive fibrogen, and impedance plethysmography, may provide confirmation.

When the thrombus fragment is released, it is rapidly swept into one of the pulmonary arteries. Very large thrombi impact in a large artery. However, the thrombus may break up and block several smaller vessels. The lower lobes are frequently involved because they have a high blood flow (see Figure 3-4).

Pulmonary infarction, that is, death of the embolized tissue, occurs infrequently. More often there is distal hemorrhage and atelectasis, but the alveolar structures remain viable. Depletion of alveolar surfactant may contribute to these changes. Infarction is more likely if the embolus completely blocks a large artery or if there is preexisting lung or heart disease. Infarction results in alveolar filling with extravasated red cells and inflammatory cells and causes opacity on the radiograph. Rarely, the infarct becomes infected, leading to an abscess. The infrequency of infarction can be explained, in part, by the fact that most emboli do not obstruct the vessel completely. In addition, bronchial artery anastomoses, and the airways supply oxygen to the lung parenchyma.

## Clinical Features

The presentation depends considerably on the size of the embolus and the patient's preexisting cardiopulmonary status.

### Medium-Sized Emboli

These often present with pleuritic pain accompanied by dyspnea, slight fever, and cough productive of blood-streaked sputum. Tachycardia is common, and on auscultation there may be a pleural friction rub. A small pleural effusion may develop. Embolism may mimic pneumonia, and recognition depends on being suspicious of the diagnosis. The chest radiograph is usually normal; a peripheral wedge-shaped shadow suggests infarction. A lung scan made after injecting radioactive albumin aggregates into the venous circulation shows one or more areas of reduced perfusion (Figure 6-7). Pulmonary angiography is diagnostic but more invasive. The distribution of ventilation, measured with radioactive gases or aerosols, is typically normal unless there is preexisting lung disease.

### Massive Emboli

These may produce sudden hemodynamic collapse with shock, pallor, central chest pain, and sometimes loss of consciousness. The pulse is rapid and weak, the blood pressure is low, and the neck veins are engorged. The electrocardiogram may show the pattern of right ventricular strain. The prognosis is variable, but some 30% of massive emboli prove fatal.

### Small Emboli

These are frequently unrecognized. However, repeated small emboli gradually obliterate the pulmonary capillary bed, resulting in pulmonary hypertension. There is prominent dyspnea on exercise, and this may lead to syncope. On examination, a right ventricular heave may be felt, and a loud pulmonary second sound may be heard. The ECG and chest radiograph confirm right ventricular hypertrophy.

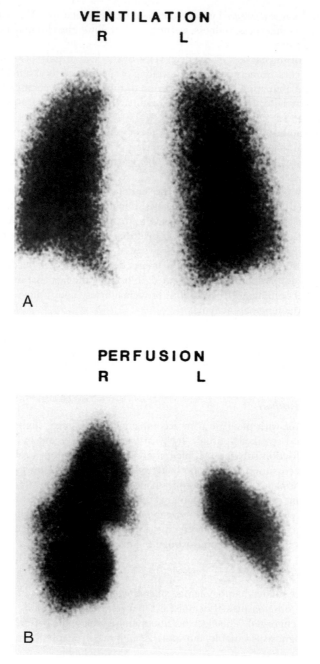

**Figure 6-7. Lung Scan in a Patient with Multiple Pulmonary Emboli. A.** The ventilation image (made with xenon-133) shows a normal pattern. **B.** The perfusion image (made with technetium-99m albumin) shows areas of absent blood flow in both lungs.

## Features of Pulmonary Embolism for Different-Sized Emboli

*Small emboli*

Frequently unrecognized

Repeated emboli may result in pulmonary hypertension

*Medium-sized emboli*

Sometimes pleuritic pain, dyspnea, slight fever

Cough may produce blood-stained sputum

May produce pleural friction rub

Chest radiograph is often normal or nearly so

Lung scan shows unperfused regions

*Massive emboli*

Hemodynamic collapse with shock, pallor, and central chest pain

Hypotension with rapid, weak pulse and neck vein engorgement

Sometimes fatal

## Pulmonary Function

### Pulmonary Circulation

This normally has a large reserve capacity because many capillaries are unfilled. When the pulmonary artery pressure rises, for example, on exercise, these capillaries are recruited and, in addition, some capillary distention occurs. This reserve means that at least half of the pulmonary circulation can be obstructed by an embolus before there is a substantial rise in pulmonary artery pressure.

In addition to the purely mechanical effects of the embolus, there is some evidence that active vasoconstriction occurs, at least for some minutes after embolization (Figure 6-8). The mechanism is not understood, but in experimental animals, local release of serotonin from platelets associated with the embolus has been implicated, as well as reflex vasoconstriction via the sympathetic nervous system. It is not known to what extent these factors operate in humans.

If the embolus is large and if the pulmonary artery pressure rises considerably, the right ventricle may begin to fail. The end-diastolic pressure increases, arrhythmias may develop, and the tricuspid valve may become incompetent. In a few cases, pulmonary edema has been seen. This is presumably caused by leakage from those capillaries not protected from the raised pulmonary artery pressure (compare high-altitude pulmonary edema).

The increase in pulmonary artery pressure gradually subsides over the subsequent days as the embolus resolves. This occurs both through fibrinolysis and through organization of the clot into a small fibrous scar attached to the vessel wall. Patency of the vessel is thus usually restored.

### Mechanics

When a pulmonary artery is occluded by a catheter in humans and experimental animals, the ventilation to that area of lung is reduced. The mechanism appears to be a direct effect of the reduced alveolar $P_{CO_2}$ on the smooth muscle of the local small airways, causing bronchoconstriction. It can be reversed by adding carbon dioxide to the inspired gas.

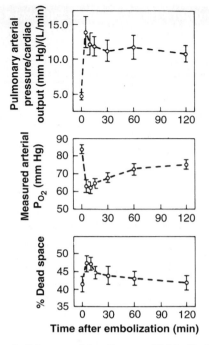

**Figure 6-8. Transient Changes in Pulmonary Artery Pressure (Related to Cardiac Output), Arterial** $P_{CO_2}$**, and Physiologic Dead Space in Dogs Following Experimental Thromboembolism.** These suggest active responses of the pulmonary circulation and airways. The importance of these mechanisms in humans is unknown. (From Dantzker DR, Wagner PD, Tornabene VW, Alzaraki NP, West JB. Gas exchange after pulmonary thromboembolization in dogs. *Circ Res* 1978L;42:92–103.)

Although this airway response to vascular obstruction is generally much weaker than the corresponding vascular response to airway obstruction (hypoxic vasoconstriction), it serves a similar homeostatic role. The reduction in airflow to the unperfused lung reduces the amount of wasted ventilation and thus the physiologic dead space. This mechanism is apparently short-lived or ineffective after pulmonary thromboembolism in humans because most measurements of the distribution of ventilation with radioactive xenon made some hours after the episode show no defect in the embolized area. However, in experimental animals, transient changes in alveolar $P_{O_2}$, physiologic dead space, and airway resistance often occur after thromboembolism (Figure 6-8).

The elastic properties of the embolized region may change some hours after the event. In experimental animals, ligation of one pulmonary artery is followed by patchy hemorrhagic edema and atelectasis in the affected lung within 24 hours. This has been attributed to the loss of pulmonary surfactant, which has a rapid turnover and apparently cannot be replenished in a lung that has lost its pulmonary blood flow. Again, it is not yet clear how often this occurs in human pulmonary thromboembolism or whether it is part of the pathological process that has been traditionally called infarction. The fact that most emboli do not completely block the vessel presumably limits its occurrence.

## Gas Exchange

Moderate hypoxemia without carbon dioxide retention is often seen after pulmonary embolism. Both the physiologic shunt and dead space are increased. Various explanations for the hypoxemia have been advanced, including diffusion impairment in areas with flows and therefore reduced transit time (see Figure 2-4), opening up of latent pulmonary artery–vein anastomoses as a consequence of the high pulmonary artery pressure and blood flow through infarcted areas.

Measurements by the multiple inert gas elimination technique show that the hypoxemia can be explained by ventilation–perfusion inequality. Figure 6-9 shows distributions from two patients after massive pulmonary embolism. The most striking features are the large shunts (blood flow to unventilated alveoli) of 20% and 39% and the existence of lung units

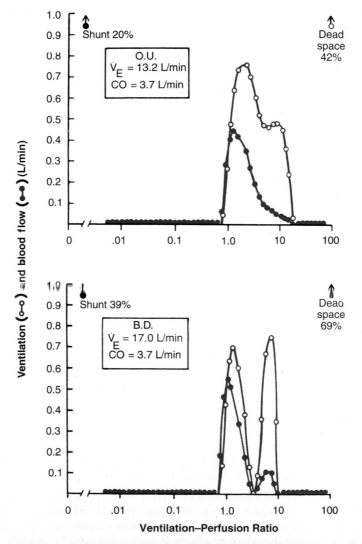

Figure 6-9. **Distributions of Ventilation–Perfusion Ratios in Two Patients with Acute Massive Pulmonary Embolism.** Note that in both instances, the hypoxemia could be explained by large shunts (blood flow to unventilated lung). In addition, there was a large increase in ventilation to lung units with abnormally high ventilation–perfusion ratios representing the embolized regions. (From D'Alonzo GE, Bower JS, DeHart P, Dantzker DR. The mechanisms of abnormal gas exchange in acute massive pulmonary embolism. *Am Rev Respir Dis* 1983;128:170–172.)

with high ventilation–perfusion ratios. The latter feature can be explained by the embolized regions where the blood flow is typically greatly reduced but not abolished completely. The precise mechanism of the shunts is not certain, but it may be blood flow through the areas of hemorrhagic atelectasis.

Sometimes, patients with pulmonary embolism also show blood flow to poorly ventilated lung units. It is of interest that in experimental thromboembolism in dogs, no true shunt is typically seen, but the hypoxemia can be explained by the increased blood flow through the nonembolized areas of lung. This results in regions with low ventilation–perfusion ratios, which depress the alveolar $P_{O_2}$. It is not clear how often this pattern occurs in human disease, but it is difficult to make many measurements in these patients because they are usually very ill.

The arterial $P_{CO_2}$ after pulmonary embolism is maintained at the normal level by increasing the ventilation to the alveoli (see Figure 2-9). The increase in ventilation may be substantial because of the large physiologic dead space, and therefore wasted ventilation, caused by the embolized areas.

Some investigators have suggested that the difference in $P_{CO_2}$ between arterial blood and end-tidal gas is a useful test for pulmonary embolism. The mixed alveolar $P_{CO_2}$ tends to be low because of the high $V_A/Q$ in the embolized region, and because there is little uneven ventilation in this disease, the end-tidal $P_{CO_2}$ is a useful measure of the mixed alveolar value.

## ▶ Pulmonary Hypertension

The normal mean pulmonary artery pressure is approximately 15 mm Hg; an increased level is called pulmonary hypertension. Three principal mechanisms are as follows:

**1.** *Increase in Left Atrial Pressure.* Examples are mitral stenosis and left ventricular failure. This is sometimes called passive pulmonary hypertension because the changes in pulmonary artery pressure are led by those in the left atrium. However, sustained increases in left atrial pressure lead to structural changes in the walls of the small pulmonary arteries, including medial hypertrophy and intimal thickening. Clinically, an increase in left atrial pressure can cause dyspnea, hemoptysis, and pulmonary edema.

**2.** *Increase in Pulmonary Blood Flow.* This occurs in congenital heart disease with left-to-right shunts through ventricular or atrial septal defects or a patent ductus arteriosus. Initially, the rise in pulmonary artery pressure is relatively small because of the ability of the pulmonary capillaries to accommodate high flows by recruitment and distension. However, sustained high flows result in structural changes in the walls of the small arteries, and eventually the pulmonary artery pressures may reach systemic levels, causing some right-to-left shunting and arterial hypoxemia.

**3.** *Increase in Pulmonary Vascular Resistance.* This is the most common cause of severe pulmonary hypertension. Again, three categories can be described:

   a. Vasoconstrictive, principally because of alveolar hypoxia as occurs at high altitude. This is also a component in the hypertension of chronic bronchitis and emphysema. Serotonin may cause transient vasoconstriction after thromboembolism, and the release of catecholamines may be a factor in some conditions, for example, neurogenic pulmonary edema. Other mediators have also been implicated, for example, in asthma (see Figure 4-18).
   b. Obstructive, as in thromboembolism. In addition, the vessels may be occluded by circulating fat, air, amniotic fluid, or cancer cells. In schistosomiasis, the parasites lodge in small arteries and cause a marked reaction.

c.  Obliterative, as in emphysema, in which the capillary bed is partly destroyed (see Figures 4-2 and 4-3). Various forms of arteritis can also occur, such as in polyarteritis nodosa. Rarely, the small veins are involved, as in pulmonary venoocclusive disease.

## Primary Pulmonary Hypertension

This is an uncommon disorder of uncertain cause, although a genetic component is recognized. Some cases may be caused by unrecognized, repeated small emboli. The majority of patients are females between 20 and 40 years old. Histologic examination of the lung shows an increase in smooth muscle in the small pulmonary arteries.

The chief symptom is dyspnea on exercise. Syncope may occur. Examination reveals signs of right ventricular hypertrophy that are confirmed by the ECG and chest radiographic appearances. Hypoxemia may be present, but ventilatory tests are usually normal. The disease typically progresses inexorably, and death occurs within a few years. If the cause is repeated thromboembolism, surgery to remove the obstruction is sometimes valuable.

## Cor Pulmonale

This term refers to right heart disease secondary to primary disease of the lung. The occurrence of right ventricular hypertrophy and fluid retention in COPD was discussed in Chapter 4. The same findings may occur late in restrictive lung disease.

The various factors that lead to pulmonary hypertension include obliteration of the capillary bed by the destruction of alveolar walls or interstitial fibrosis; obstruction by thromboemboli, hypoxic vasoconstriction, hypertrophy of smooth muscle in the walls of the small arteries; and increased viscosity of the blood caused by polycythemia. Whether the term "right heart failure" should be applied to all these patients is disputed. In some, the output of the heart is increased because it is operating high on the Starling curve, and the output can increase further on exercise. The principal physiological abnormality in these patients is fluid retention. However, in others, true failure develops. Some physicians restrict the term cor pulmonale to those patients who have ECG evidence of right ventricular hypertrophy.

## ► Pulmonary Arteriovenous Malformation

This uncommon condition is characterized by an abnormal communication between a branch of a pulmonary artery and vein. Approximately half of these patients also have telangiectases of the skin or mucous membranes, suggesting the presence of a general vascular defect. There is sometimes a family history of telangiectasia.

Small lesions cause no functional disturbances and may be found on a routine chest radiograph. Larger fistulae cause true shunts and hypoxemia. The arterial $P_{O_2}$ is depressed far below the expected value during oxygen breathing (see Figure 2.6). Sometimes a bruit can be detected over the fistula by auscultation. Finger clubbing is common.

## KEY CONCEPTS

1. Fluid movement across the pulmonary capillary endothelium is determined by the Starling equation and disturbances of the normal equilibrium can result in pulmonary edema. A common cause is an increase in capillary pressure as a result of left heart failure.

2. Clinical features of pulmonary edema include dyspnea, orthopnea, cough with blood-stained sputum, tachycardia, and rales on auscultation.

3. Two stages of pulmonary edema are recognized: interstitial and alveolar. The first is difficult to detect, but the second causes major symptoms and signs.

4. Pulmonary embolism is frequently undiagnosed. Medium-sized emboli typically cause pleuritic pain, dyspnea, and cough with blood-streaked sputum. A perfusion scan is diagnostic. Multiple small emboli can result in pulmonary hypertension.

5. Pulmonary hypertension can be caused by elevated venous pressure as in left heart failure, an increase in pulmonary blood flow as in some congenital heart diseases, or an increase in pulmonary vascular resistance as at high altitude, following thromboembolism or loss of capillaries as in emphysema.

## QUESTIONS

1. Increased movement of fluid from the lumen of pulmonary capillaries into the interstitium can be caused by:
   A. Increased permeability of the alveolar epithelial cells.
   B. Reduced capillary hydrostatic pressure.
   C. Reduced colloid osmotic pressure of the blood.
   D. Increased hydrostatic pressure in the interstitial space.
   E. Reduced colloid osmotic pressure of the interstitial fluid.

2. Concerning the blood–gas barrier in the normal lung:
   A. Fluid can drain through the interstitium of the thick side of the blood–gas barrier.
   B. The alveolar epithelium has a high permeability for water.
   C. The strength of the barrier on the thin side is mainly attributable to the endothelial cells.
   D. No protein normally crosses the capillary endothelium.
   E. Water is actively transported into the alveolar spaces by alveolar epithelial cells.

3. In the earliest stages of pulmonary edema:
   A. Fluid tracks through the interstitium of the thin side of the blood–gas barrier to the perivascular and peribronchial spaces.
   B. There is no increase in lung lymph flow.
   C. Fluid floods the alveoli one by one.
   D. The hydrostatic pressure in the interstitium probably falls.
   E. Cuffs of fluid collect around the small arteries and veins.

4. Interstitial pulmonary edema (in the absence of alveolar edema) typically results in:
   A. Septal lines on the chest radiograph.
   B. Increased lung compliance.
   C. Reduced lymph flow from the lungs.
   D. Severe hypoxemia.
   E. Fluffy shadowing on the chest radiograph.

5. When edema fluid is present in the airways and alveoli:
   A. Carbon dioxide retention typically occurs.
   B. The alveoli that contain fluid become overexpanded.
   C. The fluid is free of red blood cells.
   D. During positive pressure ventilation the fluid is moved peripherally.
   E. No changes are seen on the chest radiograph.

6. Concerning high-altitude pulmonary edema:

   A. The hypoxia directly increases capillary permeability.
   B. Pulmonary venous pressure is increased.
   C. The best treatment is to give diuretics.
   D. Dyspnea is not a feature.
   E. It Is related to the high pulmonary artery pressures caused by hypoxic vasoconstriction.

7. Concerning severe pulmonary edema with alveolar filling:

   A. Lung compliance is increased.
   B. Airway resistance is not affected.
   C. The arterial hypoxemia cannot be abolished by breathing 100% oxygen.
   D. Respiration is deep and labored.
   E. The alveolar edema causes chest pain.

8. The formation of venous thrombi is favored by:

   A. Overtransfusion with saline.
   B. Walking.
   C. Anemia.
   D. Use of oral contraceptives.
   E. Leg exercises.

9. Moderately large pulmonary emboli often cause:

   A. $CO_2$ retention.
   B. Increased physiologic dead space.
   C. Pulmonary hypotension.
   D. Rhonchi
   E. Increased cardiac output

10. Cor pulmonale:

    A. May complicate long-standing COPD.
    B. Always causes a reduced cardiac output.
    C. Does not occur in diffuse interstitial pulmonary fibrosis.
    D. Cannot cause neck vein engorgement.
    E. Cannot cause ankle edema.

# Environmental, Neoplastic, and Infectious Diseases

# 7

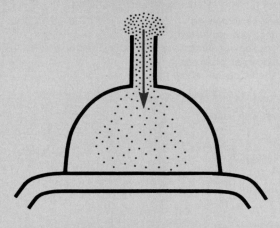

## ▶ Diseases Caused by Inhaled Particles

Many occupational and industrial lung diseases are caused by inhaled dusts. Atmospheric pollutants are also important factors in the etiology of other diseases, such as chronic bronchitis, emphysema, asthma, and bronchial carcinoma, so we will start by looking at the environment in which we all live.

## Atmospheric Pollutants

### Carbon Monoxide

This is the largest pollutant by weight in the United States (Figure 7-1, *left*). It is produced by the incomplete combustion of carbon in fuels, chiefly in the automobile engine (Figure 7-1, *right*). The main hazard of carbon monoxide is its propensity to tie up hemoglobin. Because carbon monoxide has more than 200 times the affinity of oxygen, it competes successfully with this gas. Carbon monoxide also increases the oxygen affinity of the remaining hemoglobin with the result that it does not release its oxygen so readily to the tissues. (See *Respiratory Physiology: The Essentials*, 9th ed., p. 84). A commuter using a busy urban freeway may have 5-10% of his hemoglobin bound to carbon monoxide, particularly if he is a cigarette smoker. There is evidence that this can impair mental skills. The emission of carbon monoxide and other pollutants by automobile engines can be reduced by installing a catalytic converter that processes the exhaust gases.

### Nitrogen Oxides

These are produced when fossil fuels (coal, oil) are burned at high temperatures in power stations and automobiles. These gases cause inflammation of the eyes and upper respiratory tract during smoggy conditions. At higher concentrations, they can cause acute tracheitis, acute bronchitis, and pulmonary edema. The yellow haze of smog is a result of these gases.

### Sulfur Oxides

These are corrosive, poisonous gases produced when sulfur-containing fuels are burned, chiefly by power stations. These gases cause inflammation of the mucous membranes, eyes,

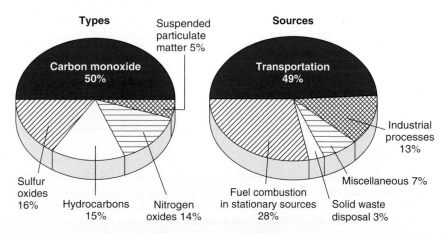

**Figure 7-1. Air Pollutants (by Weight) in the United States.** Transportation sources, especially automobiles, account for the largest amount of pollutants. Stationary sources, particularly power stations, account for 28%. (From the Environmental Protection Agency.)

upper respiratory tract, and bronchial mucosa. Short-term exposure to high concentrations causes pulmonary edema. Long-term exposure to lower levels results in chronic bronchitis in experimental animals. The best way to reduce emissions of sulfur oxides is to use low-sulfur fuels, but these are expensive.

## Hydrocarbons

Hydrocarbons, like carbon monoxide, represent unburned wasted fuel. They are not toxic at concentrations normally found in the atmosphere. However, they are hazardous because they form photochemical oxidants under the influence of sunlight (discussed later).

## Particulate Matter

This includes particles with a wide range of sizes, up to visible smoke and soot. Major sources are power stations and industrial plants. Often emission of polluting particles can be reduced by processing the waste air stream by filtering or scrubbing, although removing the smallest particles is often expensive.

## Photochemical Oxidants

These include ozone and other substances, such as peroxyacyl nitrates, aldehydes, and acrolein. They are not primary emissions but are produced by the action of sunlight on hydrocarbons and nitrogen oxides. These reactions are slow with the result that the concentration of the photochemical oxidants may increase several kilometers from where the oil was released. Photochemical oxidants cause inflammation of the eyes and respiratory tract, damage to vegetation, and offensive odors. In higher concentrations, ozone causes pulmonary edema. These oxidants contribute to the thick haze of smog.

The concentration of atmospheric pollutants is often greatly increased by a temperature inversion, that is, a low layer of cold air beneath warmer air. This prevents the normal escape of warm surface air with its pollutants to the upper atmosphere. The deleterious effects of a temperature inversion are particularly marked in a low-lying area surrounded by hills, such as the Los Angeles basin.

**Major Atmospheric Pollutants**

- Carbon monoxide
- Nitrogen oxides
- Sulfur oxides
- Hydrocarbons
- Particulate matter
- Photochemical oxidants

## Cigarette Smoke

This is one of the most important pollutants in practice because it is inhaled by devotees in concentrations many times greater than the pollutants in the atmosphere. It includes approximately 4% carbon monoxide, enough to raise the carboxyhemoglobin level in a smoker's blood to 10%. This percentage is sufficient to impair exercise and mental performance. The smoke also contains alkaloid nicotine, which stimulates the autonomic nervous system, causing tachycardia, hypertension, and sweating. Aromatic hydrocarbons and other substances, loosely called "tars," are apparently responsible for the high risk of bronchial carcinoma in cigarette smokers. A male who smokes 35 cigarettes per day has 40 times the risk of a nonsmoker. Increased risks of chronic bronchitis and emphysema and of coronary heart disease are also well documented. A single cigarette causes a marked increase in airway resistance in many smokers and nonsmokers (see Figure 3-2).

## Deposition of Aerosols in the Lung

The term *aerosol* refers to a collection of small particles that remains airborne for a substantial amount of time. Many pollutants exist in this form, and their pattern of deposition in the lung depends chiefly on their size. The properties of aerosols are also important in understanding the fate of inhaled bronchodilators. Three mechanisms of deposition are recognized.

### Impaction

*Impaction* refers to the tendency of the largest inspired particles to fail to turn the corners of the respiratory tract. As a result, many particles impinge on the mucous surfaces of the nose and pharynx (Figure 7-2A) and also on the bifurcations of the large airways. Once a particle strikes a wet surface, it is trapped and not subsequently released. The nose is remarkably efficient at removing the largest particles by this mechanism; almost all particles greater than 20 μm in diameter and approximately 95% of particles 5 μm in diameter are filtered by the nose during resting breathing. Figure 7-3 shows that most of the deposition of particles over 3 μm in diameter occurs in the nasopharynx during nose breathing.

### Sedimentation

Sedimentation is the gradual settling of particles because of their weight (Figure 7-2B). It is particularly important for medium-sized particles (1–5 μm) because the larger particles are removed by impaction and the smaller particles settle so slowly. Deposition by sedimentation occurs extensively in the small airways, including the terminal and respiratory bronchioles. The chief reason is simply that the dimensions of those airways are small and therefore the particles have a shorter distance to fall. Note that the particles, unlike gases, are not able to

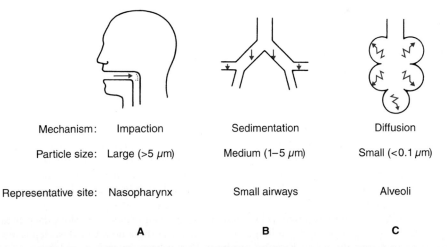

| Mechanism: | Impaction | Sedimentation | Diffusion |
|---|---|---|---|
| Particle size: | Large (>5 μm) | Medium (1–5 μm) | Small (<0.1 μm) |
| Representative site: | Nasopharynx | Small airways | Alveoli |
| | **A** | **B** | **C** |

**Figure 7-2. Scheme of Deposition of Aerosols in the Lung.** The term *representative sites* does not mean that these are the only sites where this form of deposition occurs. For example, impaction also occurs in the medium-sized bronchi, and diffusion also occurs in the large and small airways. (See text for details.)

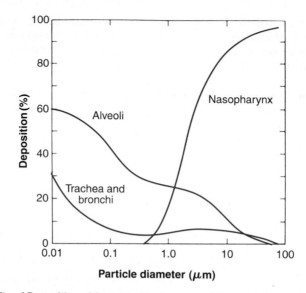

**Figure 7-3. Site of Deposition of Aerosols.** The largest particles remain in the nasopharynx, but some of the small particles can penetrate to the alveoli.

diffuse from the respiratory bronchioles to the alveoli because of their negligibly small diffusion rate. (See *Respiratory Physiology: The Essentials*, 9th ed., p. 7).

Figure 7-4 shows accumulations of dust around the terminal and respiratory bronchioles of a coal miner with early pneumoconiosis. Although the retention of dust depends on both deposition and clearance, and it is possible that some of this dust was transported from peripheral alveoli, the appearance is a graphic reminder of the vulnerability of this region of the lung. It has been suggested that some of the earliest changes in chronic bronchitis and emphysema are secondary to the deposition of atmospheric pollutants (including tobacco smoke particles) in these small airways.

## Diffusion

Diffusion is the random movement of particles as a result of their continuous bombardment by gas molecules (Figure 7-2C). It occurs to a significant extent only in the smallest particles (less than 0.1 μm in diameter). Deposition by diffusion chiefly takes place in the small airways and alveoli where the distances to the wall are least. However, some deposition by this mechanism also occurs in the larger airways.

Many inhaled particles are not deposited at all but are exhaled with the next breath. In fact, only some 30% of 0.5 μm particles may be left in the lung during normal resting breathing. These particles are too small to impact or sediment to a large extent. In addition, they are too large to diffuse significantly. As a result, they do not move from the terminal and respiratory bronchioles to the alveoli by diffusion, which is the normal mode of gas movement in this region. Small particles may become larger during inspiration by aggregation or by absorbing water.

The pattern of ventilation affects the amount of aerosol deposition. Slow, deep breaths increase the penetration into the lung and thus increase the amount of dust deposited by sedimentation and diffusion. Exercise results in higher rates of airflow and it particularly increases deposition by impaction. In general, deposition of dust is proportional to the ventilation during exercise, which is therefore an important factor during work at the coalface, for example.

## Deposition and Clearance of Inhaled Particles

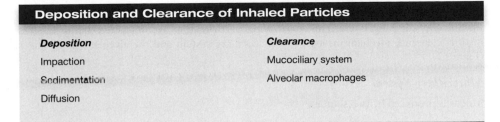

| *Deposition* | *Clearance* |
| --- | --- |
| Impaction | Mucociliary system |
| Sedimentation | Alveolar macrophages |
| Diffusion | |

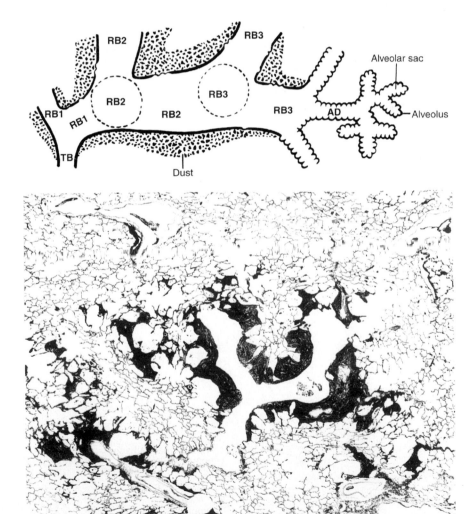

**Figure 7-4. Section of Lung from a Coal Miner Showing Accumulations of Dust Around the Respiratory Bronchioles.** These small airways show some dilatation, sometimes called focal emphysema. (From Heppleston AG, Leopold JG. Chronic pulmonary emphysema: Anatomy and pathogenesis. *Am J Med* 1961;31:279–291.)

## Clearance of Deposited Particles

Fortunately, the lung is efficient at removing particles that are deposited within it. Two distinct clearance mechanisms exist: the mucociliary system and the alveolar macrophages (Figure 7-5).

### Mucociliary System

Mucus is produced by two sources:

**1.** Bronchial seromucous glands situated deep in the bronchial walls (see Figures 4-6, 4-7, and 7-6). Both mucus-producing and serous-producing cells are present, and ducts lead the mucus to the airway surface.

**2.** Goblet cells, which form part of the bronchial epithelium.

The normal mucus film is approximately 5- to 10-μm thick and has two layers (Figure 7-6). The superficial gel layer is relatively tenacious and viscous. As a result, it is efficient at trapping deposited particles. The deeper sol layer is less viscous and thus allows the cilia to beat within it easily. It is likely that the abnormal retention of secretions that occurs in some diseases is caused by changes in the composition of the mucus, with the result that it cannot be propelled easily by the cilia.

The mucus contains the immunoglobulin IgA, which is derived from plasma cells and lymphoid tissue. This humoral factor is an important defense against foreign proteins, bacteria, and viruses.

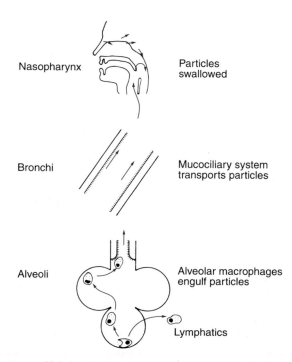

**Figure 7-5. Clearance of Inhaled Particles from the Lung.** Particles that deposit on the surface of the airways are transported by the mucociliary escalator and swallowed. Particles that reach the alveoli are engulfed by macrophages, which either migrate to the ciliary surface or escape via the lymphatics.

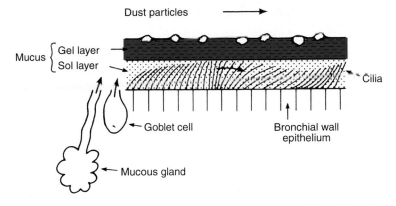

**Figure 7-6. Mucociliary Escalator.** The mucous film consists of a superficial gel layer that traps inhaled particles and a deeper sol layer. It is propelled by cilia.

The cilia are 5- to 7-μm long and beat in a synchronized fashion at between 1000 and 1500 times per minute. During the forward stroke, the tips of the cilia apparently come in contact with the gel layer, thus propelling it. However, during the recovery phase, the cilia are bent so much that they move entirely within the sol layer, where the resistance is less.

The mucous blanket moves up at around 1 mm/min in small peripheral airways but as fast as 2 cm/min in the trachea, and eventually the particles reach the level of the pharynx where they are swallowed. The clearance of a healthy bronchial mucosa is essentially complete in less than 24 hours. In very dusty environments, mucous secretion may be increased so much that cough and expectoration assist in the clearance.

The normal operation of the mucociliary system is affected by pollution and disease. The cilia apparently can be paralyzed by the inhalation of toxic gases, such as oxides of sulfur and nitrogen, and perhaps by tobacco smoke. In acute inflammation of the respiratory tract, the bronchial epithelium may be denuded. Changes in the character of the mucus may occur with infection, thus making it difficult for the cilia to transport it. Mucous plugging of bronchi occurs in asthma, but the mechanism is unknown. Finally, in chronic infections such as bronchiectasis and chronic bronchitis, the volume of secretions may be so great that the ciliary transport system is overwhelmed.

### Alveolar Macrophages

The mucociliary system stops short of the alveoli, and particles deposited there are engulfed by macrophages. These amoeboid cells roam around the surface of the alveoli. When they phagocytose foreign particles, they either migrate to the small airways where they load on to the mucociliary escalator (Figure 7-5) or they leave the lung in the lymphatics or possibly the blood. When the dust burden is large or the dust particles are toxic, some of the macrophages migrate through the walls of the respiratory bronchioles and dump their dust there. Figure 7-4 shows the accumulations of dust around the respiratory bronchioles in the lung of a coal miner. If the dust is toxic, such as silica, a fibrous reaction is stimulated in this region.

The macrophages not only transport bacteria out of the lung but also kill them in situ by means of the lysozymes they contain. As a consequence, the alveoli quickly become sterile, although it takes some time for the dead organisms to be cleared from the lung. Immunologic mechanisms are also important in the antibacterial action of macrophages.

Normal macrophage activity can be impaired by various factors, such as cigarette smoke, oxidant gases such as ozone, alveolar hypoxia, radiation, the administration of corticosteroids, and the ingestion of alcohol. Macrophages that engulf particles of silica are often destroyed by this toxic material.

## Coal Workers' Pneumoconiosis

The term *pneumoconiosis* refers to parenchymal lung disease caused by inorganic dust inhalation. One form seen in coal workers is directly related to the amount of coal dust to which the miner has been exposed.

### Pathology

Early and late forms of the disease should be distinguished. In simple pneumoconiosis, there are aggregations of coal particles around terminal and respiratory bronchioles, with some dilatation of these small airways (Figure 7-4). In the advanced form of the disease, known as progressive massive fibrosis, condensed masses of black fibrous tissue infiltrated with dust are seen. Only a small fraction of miners exposed to heavy dust concentrations develop progressive massive fibrosis.

### Clinical Features

Simple pneumoconiosis apparently causes little disability despite its radiographic appearances. The dyspnea and cough that often accompany the disease are closely related to the smoking history of the miner and are probably chiefly caused by associated chronic bronchitis and emphysema. By contrast, progressive massive fibrosis usually causes increasing dyspnea and may terminate in respiratory failure.

The chest radiograph of simple pneumoconiosis shows a delicate micronodular mottling, and various stages in the advance of the disease are recognized depending on the density of the shadows. Progressive massive fibrosis results in large, irregular dense opacities often surrounded by abnormally radiolucent lung.

### Pulmonary Function

Simple pneumoconiosis usually causes little functional impairment by itself. However, sometimes a small reduction in forced expiratory volume, a rise in residual volume, and a fall in arterial $P_{O_2}$ are seen. It is often difficult to know whether these changes are caused by associated chronic bronchitis and emphysema.

Progressive massive fibrosis causes a mixed obstructive and restrictive pattern. Distortion of the airways results in irreversible obstructive changes, whereas the large masses of fibrous tissue reduce the useful volume of the lung. Increasing hypoxemia, cor pulmonale, and terminal respiratory failure may occur.

## Silicosis

This pneumoconiosis is caused by the inhalation of silica ($SiO_2$) during quarrying, mining, or sandblasting. Whereas coal dust is virtually inert, silica particles are toxic and provoke a severe fibrous reaction in the lung.

### Pathology

Silicotic nodules composed of concentric whorls of dense collagen fibers are found around respiratory bronchioles, inside alveoli, and along the lymphatics. Silica particles may be seen in the nodules.

### Clinical Features

Mild forms of the disease may cause no symptoms, although the chest radiograph shows fine nodular markings. Advanced disease results in cough and severe dyspnea, especially on exercise. The radiograph sometimes shows streaks of fibrous tissue, and progressive massive fibrosis may develop. The disease may progress long after exposure to the dust has ceased. There is an increased risk of pulmonary tuberculosis.

### Pulmonary Function

The changes are similar to those seen in coal workers' pneumoconiosis but are often more severe. In advanced disease, generalized interstitial fibrosis may develop, with a restrictive type of defect, severe dyspnea and hypoxemia on exercise, and a reduced diffusing capacity.

## Asbestos-Related Diseases

Asbestos is a naturally occurring fibrous mineral silicate that is used in a variety of industrial applications, including heat insulation, pipe lagging, roofing materials, and brake linings. Asbestos fibers are long and thin, and it is possible that their aerodynamic characteristics allow them to penetrate far into the lung. When they are in the lung, they may become encased in proteinaceous material. If these are coughed up in the sputum, they are known as asbestos bodies.

Three health hazards are recognized:

**1.** Diffuse interstitial fibrosis (asbestosis) may gradually occur after heavy exposure. There is a progressive dyspnea (especially on exercise), weakness, and finger clubbing. On auscultation, there are fine basal crepitations. The chest radiograph shows haziness or mottling. Pulmonary function tests in advanced disease reveal a typical restrictive pattern with reductions of vital capacity and lung compliance. A fall in diffusing capacity occurs relatively early in the disease.

**2.** Bronchial carcinoma is a common complication. Cigarette smoking is often an aggravating factor.

**3.** Pleural disease may occur after trivial exposure, for example, in a person who washes the clothes of an asbestos worker. Pleural thickening and plaques are common but are usually harmless. Malignant mesothelioma may develop as much as 40 years after light exposure. It causes progressive restriction of chest movement, severe chest pain, and a rapid downhill course.

## Other Pneumoconioses

A variety of other dusts cause simple pneumoconiosis. Examples include iron and its oxides, which cause siderosis and result in a striking, mottled radiographic appearance. Antimony and tin are other culprits. Beryllium exposure results in granulomatous lesions of acute or chronic types. The latter results in interstitial fibrosis with its typical restrictive pattern of dysfunction. The disease is now much less common than it was as a result of strict control of beryllium in industry.

## Byssinosis

Some inhaled organic dusts cause airway reactions rather than alveolar reactions. A good example is byssinosis, which follows exposure to cotton dust, especially in the cardroom where the fibers are initially processed.

The pathogenesis is not fully understood, but it appears that the inhalation of some active component in the bracts (leaves around the stem of the cotton boll) leads to the release of histamine from mast cells in the lung. The resulting bronchoconstriction causes dyspnea and wheezing. A feature of the disease is that the symptoms are worse on entering the mill, especially after a period of absence. For this reason it is sometimes known as

"Monday fever." The symptoms include dyspnea, tightness of the chest, wheezing, and an irritating cough. Workers who have already had chronic bronchitis or asthma are especially susceptible.

Pulmonary function tests show an obstructive pattern with reductions in $FEV_1$, $FEV/FVC$ %, $FEF_{25-75\%}$, and FVC. Airway resistance is increased and the amount of inequality of ventilation rises after exposure. Typically, these abnormalities gradually become worse over the course of the working day, but partial or complete recovery occurs during the night or over the weekend. There is no evidence of parenchymal involvement, and the chest radiograph is normal. However, epidemiologic studies show that daily exposure over 20 years or so causes permanent impairment of lung function of the type associated with COPD.

## Occupational Asthma

Various occupations involve exposure to allergenic organic dusts, and some individuals develop hypersensitivity. These individuals include flour mill workers who are sensitive to the wheat weevil, printers exposed to gum acacia, and workers handling fur or feathers. Toluene diisocyanate (TDI) is a special case because some individuals develop an extreme sensitivity to this substance, which is used in the manufacture of polyurethane products.

## ▶ Neoplastic Diseases

## Bronchial Carcinoma

This book is about the function of the diseased lung and how this is measured using pulmonary function tests. For neoplastic diseases, this is generally not an important topic because the effects on pulmonary function are minor in the context of diagnosis, staging, and treatment. In general the physician's objective is to diagnose the carcinoma early enough to remove it surgically. Pulmonary function tests are almost never of value in this regard. However, lung function is often impaired in moderately advanced disease where surgical removal is usually not an option. Accordingly, this section is relatively brief, and textbooks of pathology or internal medicine should be consulted for additional details on diagnosis, staging, and management of this disease.

The incidence of the disease is awesome; around 30% of male and 25% of female cancer deaths are from lung cancer. Much of this disease is preventable.

### Pathogenesis

There is overwhelming evidence that cigarette smoking is a major factor. Epidemiologic studies show that an individual who smokes 20 cigarettes a day has about 20 times the chance of dying from the disease than a nonsmoker of the same age and sex. Furthermore, the risk decreases dramatically if the individual stops smoking.

The specific causative agents in cigarette smoke are uncertain, but many potential carcinogenic substances are present, including aromatic hydrocarbons, phenols, and radioisotopes. Many smoke particles are submicronic and penetrate far into the lung. However, the fact that many bronchogenic carcinomas originate in the large bronchi suggests that deposition by impaction or sedimentation may play an important role (Figure 7-2). Also, the large bronchi are exposed to a high concentration of tobacco smoke products as the material is transported from the more peripheral regions by the mucociliary system. Individuals who inhale other peoples' smoke (passive smokers) have an increased risk.

Other etiological factors are recognized. Urban dwellers are more at risk, suggesting that atmospheric pollution plays a part. This finding is hardly surprising in view of the variety of chronic respiratory tract irritants that exist in city air (Figure 7-1). Occupational factors also exist, especially exposure to chromates, nickel, arsenic, asbestos, and radioactive gases.

## Classification

Most pulmonary neoplasms can be divided into small-cell and non–small-cell types.

**A.** *Small-cell carcinomas.* These contain a homogeneous population of oatlike cells giving a characteristic appearance. Up to one-third of all neoplasms are of this type. They are highly malignant with rapid dissemination. These tumors are seldom seen in peripheral lung and usually do not cavitate.

**B.** *Non–small-cell carcinomas.* There are four main types.

**1.** *Squamous carcinomas* are the most common and account for nearly half of all cases. Microscopically, intercellular bridges are visible, keratin is present, and the cells often form a whorl or nest pattern. Cavitation occurs sometimes. There is often an initial response to radiation but not to chemotherapy.

**2.** *Large-cell carcinomas* contain cells of approximately the same size as squamous carcinomas but the characteristic whorls are not seen. They tend to occur in the periphery of the lung. Approximately 10% of neoplasms are in this category.

**3.** *Adenocarcinomas* show glandular differentiation and often produce mucus. They typically occur peripherally, and the incidence of occurrence appears to be increasing and is greatest in women.

**4.** *Bronchioalveolar carcinomas* are a subtype of adenocarcinoma that arise from type II alveolar cells and are rare. They are not related to smoking.

Many tumors show some heterogeneity of cell type, thus making classification difficult. Also, there are a number of other neoplastic diseases of the lung.

## Clinical Features

An unproductive cough or hemoptysis is a common early symptom. Sometimes hoarseness is the first clue and is caused by involvement of the left recurrent laryngeal nerve. Dyspnea caused by pleural effusion or bronchial obstruction, and chest pain caused by pleural involvement, usually are late symptoms. Examination of the chest is often negative, although signs of lobar collapse or consolidation may be found. The chest radiograph is often crucial, but a small carcinoma may not be visible. Bronchoscopy and sputum cytology are valuable aids to early diagnosis.

## Pulmonary Function

As stated earlier, the physician's objective is to diagnose a carcinoma of the bronchus early enough to remove it surgically. Pulmonary function tests are rarely of value in this regard. However, lung function is often impaired in moderately advanced disease.

A large pleural effusion causes a restrictive defect, as may the collapse of a lobe after complete bronchial obstruction. Partial obstruction of a large bronchus can result in an obstructive pattern. The obstruction can be caused either by a tumor of the bronchial wall or by compression by an enlarged lymph gland. Sometimes the movement of the lung on the affected side is seen to lag behind the normal lung, and air may cycle back and forth between the normal and obstructed lobes (see *Respiratory Physiology: The Essentials*, 9th ed., p. 174). This cycle is known as pendelluft (swinging air). Complete obstruction of a mainstem bronchus can give a pseudorestrictive pattern because half the lung is not ventilating. Partial or complete bronchial obstruction usually causes some hypoxemia.

## ▶  Infectious Diseases

Infectious diseases are of great importance in pulmonary medicine. However they generally do not cause specific patterns of impaired pulmonary function, and pulmonary function tests are of little value in the diagnosis or management of these patients. Since this book is about the function of the diseased lung and its measurement using pulmonary function tests, infectious diseases do not merit much prominence. A textbook on internal medicine or pathology should be consulted for further details.

## Pneumonia

This term refers to inflammation of the lung parenchyma associated with alveolar filling by exudate.

### Pathology

The alveoli are crammed with cells, chiefly polymorphonuclear leukocytes. Resolution often occurs with restoration of the normal morphology. However, suppuration may result in necrosis of tissue, causing a lung abscess. Special forms of pneumonia include that, following aspiration of gastric fluid or animal or mineral oil (lipoid pneumonia). Psittacosis is a form transmitted from infected parrots by a rickettsia.

### Clinical Features

These features vary considerably depending on the causative organism, the age of the patient, and his or her general condition. The usual features include malaise, fever, and cough. Pleuritic pain is common and is worse on deep breathing. Examination reveals rapid shallow breathing, tachycardia, and sometimes cyanosis. Often there are signs of consolidation, and the chest radiograph shows opacification. This may involve all of a lobe (lobar pneumonia), but frequently the distribution is patchy (bronchopneumonia). Sputum examination and culture frequently identify the causative organism.

### Pulmonary Function

Because the pneumonic region is not ventilated, it causes shunting and hypoxemia. The severity of these conditions depends on the local pulmonary blood flow, which may be substantially reduced either by the disease process itself or by hypoxic vasoconstriction. However, patients with severe pneumonia may be cyanosed. Carbon dioxide retention does not generally occur. Chest movement may be restricted by pleural pain or by a pleural effusion.

## Tuberculosis

Pulmonary tuberculosis takes many forms. Early lesions do not affect pulmonary function, but in the late stages of the disease, severe functional impairment may occur, leading to respiratory failure. Advanced disease is much less common now because of treatment with antituberculous drugs.

The initial infection results in a primary complex with hilar lymph node enlargement. This enlargement rapidly resolves and is usually not recognized. The postprimary infection is usually in the apices of the lungs, apparently because of the high ventilation–perfusion ratio there, and the resulting high $P_{O_2}$ (see Figure 3-4) provide a favorable environment for the growth of the bacillus. If this infection heals, as it generally does, no functional impairment results.

Extension of the infection may cause pneumonia, miliary infection, cavitation, lobar collapse, or pleural effusion. Ultimately, severe fibrosis may develop, with restrictive impairment of function. The treatment of tuberculosis is now so effective that the disease is less often seen in well-developed countries. However, the emergence of strains resistant to antibiotics is a problem. The disease is still a major problem in underdeveloped countries and may therefore occur in immigrants. In addition, immune-compromised patients, for example those with acquired immunodeficiency syndrome (AIDS), can develop florid forms.

## Fungus Infections

*Histoplasmosis* is the most common fungus in the United States. In most adults it does not cause symptoms but occasionally it results in calcification which is readily detected on a radiograph. *Coccidiodomycosis* is common in the San Joaquin Valley of California where the majority of people have a positive skin test. Many cases are asymptomatic, but some develop a fever with cough. The fungus of *candidiasis* is a normal inhabitant of the mouth and gastrointestinal tract and this disease is common but usually benign.

## Pulmonary Involvement in AIDS

AIDS frequently involves the lung. The most common infection is *Pneumocystis carinii*, but *Mycobacterium avium-intracellulare* and cytomegalovirus infections also occur frequently. Less frequent infections include tuberculosis and *Legionella*. Kaposi's sarcoma may occur in the lung. In patients from high-risk groups who present with these pulmonary problems, AIDS should be suspected.

## ▶ Suppurative Diseases

## Bronchiectasis

This disease is characterized by dilatation of bronchi with local suppuration.

### *Pathology*

The mucosal surface of the affected bronchi shows loss of ciliated epithelium, squamous metaplasia, and infiltration with inflammatory cells. Pus is present in the lumen during infective exacerbations. The surrounding lung often shows fibrosis and old inflammatory changes.

### *Clinical Features*

The disease usually follows childhood pneumonia, and the prevalence has fallen greatly since the introduction of powerful antibiotics. The cardinal feature is a productive cough with yellow or green sputum. This sputum may occur only after a cold or it may be present continuously. There may be hemoptysis and halitosis. Crepitations are often heard, and finger clubbing is seen in severe cases. The chest radiograph shows increased markings.

### *Pulmonary Function*

Mild disease causes no loss of function. In more advanced cases, there is a reduction of FEV and FVC because of chronic inflammatory changes, including fibrosis. Radioactive isotope measurements show reduced ventilation and pulmonary blood flow in the affected area, but there may be a greatly increased bronchial artery supply to the diseased tissue. Hypoxemia may develop as a result of blood flow through unventilated lung.

## Cystic Fibrosis

This is a disease of all exocrine glands caused by a genetic abnormality affecting chloride and sodium transport. In the lung, it takes the form of bronchiectasis and bronchiolitis.

Identification of the specific genetic defect has raised the possibility of effective gene therapy, but this has not proved possible to date.

## Pathology

The principal organ affected is the pancreas, where the tissue atrophies and the ducts remain as dilated cysts. In the lung there are excessive secretions from the hypertrophied mucous glands. Ciliary activity is also apparently impaired, and mucous plugging of small airways and chronic infection follow. Malnutrition secondary to pancreatic failure may lower resistance to infection.

## Clinical Features

A few patients die of meconium ileus shortly after birth, and others remain small and malnourished. The respiratory symptoms include productive cough, frequent chest infections, and decreased exercise tolerance. Finger clubbing is often prominent. Auscultation may reveal coarse rales and rhonchi. The chest radiograph is abnormal early in the disease and shows areas of consolidation, fibrosis, and cystic changes. In young children, the finding of a high sodium concentration in the sweat confirms the diagnosis.

Until recently, death almost invariably occurred before adulthood among patients with cystic fibrosis, but with improved treatment of chest infections, survival into the 20s or beyond is now increasingly seen. Indeed, the disease should be considered when a teenager or a young adult presents with features of chronic bronchitis.

## Pulmonary Function

An abnormal distribution of ventilation and an increased alveolar–arterial $O_2$ difference are early changes. Some investigators report that tests of small-airway function, such as flow rates at low lung volumes, may detect minimal disease. There are decreases in $FEV_1$ and $FEF_{25-75\%}$ that do not respond to bronchodilators. RV and FRC are raised and there may be loss of elastic recoil. Exercise tolerance falls as the disease progresses.

## KEY CONCEPTS

1. The most important atmospheric pollutants include carbon monoxide, oxides of nitrogen and sulfur, hydrocarbons, particulates, and photochemical oxidants.

2. Most pollutants occur as aerosols and are deposited in the lung by impaction, sedimentation, or diffusion.

3. Deposited pollutants are removed by the mucociliary system in the airways and macrophages in the alveoli.

4. Coal workers' pneumoconiosis results from long-term exposure to coal dust. In its mild form it causes dyspnea and cough together with mottling of the chest radiograph, but sometimes the role of chronic bronchitis in the symptoms is difficult to differentiate in a smoker.

5. Other pneumoconioses include asbestos-related diseases. Byssinosis is caused by organic cotton dust. Occupational asthma also occurs in some industries.

6. Infectious diseases of the lung are common and important but generally do not require pulmonary function tests. Pneumonia particularly affects the elderly and generally responds well to antibiotics. Pulmonary tuberculosis is a scourge in underdeveloped countries and is also seen in immune-compromised patients anywhere. Resistance to antibiotics is increasingly common.

7. Bronchial carcinoma is largely caused by cigarette smoking and accounts for about 30% of male cancer deaths. Although various types are recognized, the prognosis is often very poor.

8. Cystic fibrosis is a genetic abnormality of all exocrine glands, and in the lung causes bronchitis and bronchiectasis. Good medical treatment has greatly increased the lifespan of these patients.

## QUESTIONS

1. Which of the following atmospheric pollutants is present in the highest concentration (by weight) in the United States?
   A. Hydrocarbons.
   B. Sulfur oxides.
   C. Nitrogen oxides.
   D. Carbon monoxide.
   E. Ozone.

2. Concerning smog:
   A. Ozone is mainly produced in automobile engines.
   B. A temperature inversion occurs when the air near the ground is hotter than the air above.
   C. The main source of sulfur oxides is the automobile.
   D. Nitrogen oxides can cause inflammation of the upper respiratory tract.
   E. Scrubbing flue gases is ineffective in removing particulates.

3. Concerning cigarette smoke:
   A. Inhaled smoke contains negligible amounts of carbon monoxide.
   B. Cigarette smokers can have enough carboxyhemoglobin level in their blood to impair mental skills.
   C. Nicotine is not addictive.
   D. The risk of coronary heart disease is not affected by smoking.
   E. The concentration of pollutants in cigarette smoke is less than in the air of a large city on a smoggy day.

4. Concerning the deposition of aerosol in the lung:
   A. Most particles less than 5 μm in diameter are filtered by the nose during resting breathing.
   B. Many inhaled particles are deposited in the region of the terminal and respiratory bronchioles.
   C. Astronauts who are weightless have the same particle deposition as when they are on earth.
   D. Particles 0.5 μm diameter diffuse almost as fast as gas molecules.
   E. Many particles larger than 10 μm diameter are not deposited in the lung but are exhaled with the next breath.

5. In a coal miner, the deposition of coal dust in the lung will be reduced by:
   A. Frequent coughing.
   B. Exercise.
   C. Mining operations that produce very small dust particles.
   D. Rapid deep breathing.
   E. Nose breathing, as opposed to mouth breathing.

6. Concerning the mucociliary escalator in the lung:
   A. Most of the mucus comes from goblet cells in the epithelium.
   B. Trapped particles move more slowly in the trachea than in the peripheral airways.
   C. Normal clearances take several days.
   D. The cilia beat about twice a second.
   E. The composition of the mucous film is altered in some diseases.

7. Pneumonia:
    A. Usually leaves a large fibrotic scar in the affected lung.
    B. Never causes chest pain.
    C. Can result in hypoxemia.
    D. Is not associated with fever.
    E. Does not cause coughing.

8. Concerning bronchial carcinoma:
    A. The disease is more common in females than males.
    B. The specific carcinogenic agent in cigarette smoke is known.
    C. Pulmonary function tests are important in the early detection of the disease.
    D. Small cell carcinomas are the most common type.
    E. A carcinoma is always visible on a good chest radiograph.

9. Concerning cystic fibrosis:
    A. The disease is confined to the lungs.
    B. It is rare for affected children to survive until the age of 20.
    C. Finger clubbing is not seen.
    D. The composition of the sweat is normal.
    E. The gene responsible for the disease has been identified.

# PART THREE

# Function of the Failing Lung

Respiratory failure is the result of many types of acute or chronic lung disease. Part Three is devoted to the physiologic principles of respiratory failure and its chief modes of treatment: oxygen administration and mechanical ventilation.

# Respiratory Failure

8

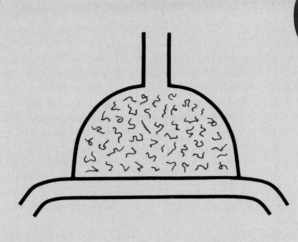

Respiratory failure is said to occur when the lung fails to oxygenate the arterial blood adequately and/or fails to prevent $CO_2$ retention. There is no absolute definition of the levels of arterial $P_{O_2}$ and $P_{CO_2}$ that indicate respiratory failure. However, a $P_{O_2}$ of less than 60 mm Hg or a $P_{CO_2}$ of more than 50 mm Hg are numbers that are often quoted. In practice, the significance of such values depends considerably on the patient's history.

## ▶ Gas Exchange in Respiratory Failure

### Patterns of Arterial Blood Gases

Various types of respiratory failure are associated with different degrees of hypoxemia and $CO_2$ retention. Figure 8-1 shows an $O_2$–$CO_2$ diagram (see *Respiratory Physiology: The Essentials*, 9th ed., pp. 68 and 170) with the line for a respiratory exchange ratio of 0.8. Pure *hypoventilation* leading to respiratory failure moves the arterial $P_{O_2}$ and $P_{CO_2}$ in the direction indicated by arrow A. This pattern occurs in respiratory failure caused by neuromuscular disease, such as poliomyelitis, or by an overdose of a narcotic drug (see Figures 2-2 and 2-3). Severe *ventilation–perfusion ratio inequality* with alveolar ventilation inadequate to maintain a normal arterial $P_{CO_2}$ results in movement along a line, such as B. The hypoxemia is more severe in relation to the hypercapnia than in the case of pure hypoventilation. Such a pattern is frequently seen in the respiratory failure of chronic obstructive pulmonary disease (COPD).

Severe interstitial disease sometimes results in movement along line C. Here there is increasingly severe hypoxemia but no $CO_2$ retention because of the raised ventilation. This pattern may be seen in advanced diffuse interstitial lung disease or sarcoidosis. Sometimes there is a rise in arterial $P_{CO_2}$, but this is typically less marked than in obstructive diseases.

In respiratory failure caused by the adult respiratory distress syndrome (ARDS), the arterial $P_{CO_2}$ may be low, as shown by line D, but the hypoxemia may be extreme. Such patients are usually treated with added inspired oxygen, which raises the arterial $P_{O_2}$ but often does not affect the $P_{CO_2}$ (D to E), although in some instances $P_{CO_2}$ may rise. Oxygen therapy to patients whose respiratory failure is caused by COPD improves the arterial $P_{O_2}$ but frequently causes a rise in $P_{CO_2}$ because of depression of ventilation (B to F).

### Hypoxemia of Respiratory Failure

#### Causes

Any of the four mechanisms of hypoxemia—hypoventilation, diffusion impairment, shunt, and ventilation–perfusion inequality—can contribute to the severe hypoxemia of respiratory failure. However, the most important cause by far is ventilation–perfusion inequality

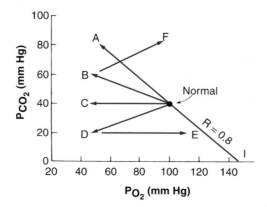

**Figure 8-1. Patterns of Arterial $P_{O_2}$ and $P_{CO_2}$ in Different Types of Respiratory Failure.** Note that the $P_{CO_2}$ can be high, as in pure hypoventilation (*line A*), or low, as in ARDS (*line D*). The broken lines show the effects of oxygen breathing. (See text for further details.)

(including blood flow through unventilated lung). This mechanism is largely responsible for the low arterial $P_{O_2}$ in respiratory failure complicating obstructive diseases, restrictive diseases, and ARDS.

## Detection

Severe hypoxemia causes cyanosis, cardiovascular signs such as tachycardia, and central nervous system effects such as mental confusion. However, a discussion of the detection of hypoxemia from these signs is largely academic because measurement of the $P_{O_2}$ in the arterial blood is essential in determining the degree of hypoxemia in patients with suspected respiratory failure.

## Tissue Hypoxia

Hypoxemia is dangerous because it causes tissue hypoxia. However, the arterial $P_{O_2}$ is only one factor in the delivery of oxygen to the tissues. Other factors include the oxygen capacity of the blood, the oxygen affinity of the hemoglobin, cardiac output, and the distribution of blood flow.

Tissues vary considerably in their vulnerability to hypoxia. Those at greatest risk include the central nervous system and the myocardium. Cessation of blood flow to the cerebral cortex results in loss of function within 4 to 6 seconds, loss of consciousness in 10 to 20 seconds, and irreversible changes in 3 to 5 minutes.

If the $P_{O_2}$ in tissue falls below a critical level, aerobic oxidation ceases and anaerobic glycolysis takes over with the formation and release of increasing amounts of lactic acid. The $P_{O_2}$ at which this occurs is not accurately known and probably varies among tissues. However, there is evidence that the critical intracellular $P_{O_2}$ is of the order of 1–3 mm Hg in the region of the mitochondria.

Anaerobic glycolysis is a relatively inefficient method of obtaining energy from glucose. Nevertheless, it plays a critical role in maintaining tissue viability in respiratory failure. The large amounts of lactic acid that are formed are released into the blood, causing a metabolic acidosis. If tissue oxygenation subsequently improves, the lactic acid can be reconverted to glucose or used directly for energy. Most of this reconversion takes place in the liver.

## Effects of Severe Hypoxemia

Mild hypoxemia produces few physiologic changes. It should be recalled that the arterial oxygen saturation is still approximately 90% when the $P_{O_2}$ is only 60 mm Hg at a normal pH (see Figure 2-1). The only abnormalities are a slight impairment of mental performance, diminished visual acuity, and perhaps mild hyperventilation.

When the arterial $P_{O_2}$ drops quickly below 40-50 mm Hg, deleterious effects are seen in several organ systems. The central nervous system is particularly vulnerable, and the patient often has headache, somnolence, or clouding of consciousness. Profound acute hypoxemia may cause convulsions, retinal hemorrhages, and permanent brain damage. The cardiovascular system shows tachycardia and mild hypertension, partly caused by the release of catecholamines; in severe hypoxemia there may be bradycardia and hypotension. Signs of heart failure may occur if there is associated coronary artery disease. Renal function is impaired, and sodium retention and proteinuria may be seen. Pulmonary hypertension is common because of the associated alveolar hypoxia.

# Hypercapnia in Respiratory Failure

## Causes

Both mechanisms of $CO_2$ retention—hypoventilation and ventilation–perfusion inequality—can be important in respiratory failure. Hypoventilation is the cause in respiratory failure resulting from neuromuscular diseases such as the Guillain-Barré syndrome, drug over-dose such as barbiturate poisoning, or a chest wall abnormality such as crushed chest (see Figure 2-3 and Table 2-1). Ventilation–perfusion inequality is the culprit in severe COPD and long-standing interstitial disease.

An important cause of $CO_2$ retention in respiratory failure is the injudicious use of oxygen therapy. Many patients with COPD gradually develop severe hypoxemia and some $CO_2$ retention over a period of months. It is not customary to refer to this situation as respiratory failure because these patients can continue in this state for long periods. However, such a patient usually has a high work of breathing (see Figure 4-13), and much of the ventilatory drive comes from hypoxic stimulation of the peripheral chemoreceptors. The arterial pH is nearly normal because of renal retention of bicarbonate (compensated respiratory acidosis), and the pH of the cerebrospinal fluid (CSF) is also nearly normal because of an increase in bicarbonate there. Thus, despite an increased arterial $P_{CO_2}$, the main ventilatory drive comes from the hypoxemia.

If this patient develops a relatively mild intercurrent respiratory infection and is treated with a high inspired oxygen concentration, a dangerous situation can rapidly develop. The hypoxic ventilatory drive may be abolished while the work of breathing is increased because of retained secretions or bronchospasm. As a result, the ventilation may become grossly depressed and high levels of arterial $P_{CO_2}$ may develop. In addition, profound hypoxemia may ensue if the oxygen is discontinued. This is because even if the ventilation does return to its previous level, the patient may take many minutes to unload the large accumulation of $CO_2$ in the tissues because of the large body stores of this gas.

A secondary cause of $CO_2$ retention in these patients may be the release of hypoxic vasoconstriction in poorly ventilated areas of lung as a result of the increased alveolar $P_{CO_2}$. The consequences of this are increased blood flow to low $\dot{V}_A/\dot{Q}$ areas and a worsening of $\dot{V}_A/\dot{Q}$ inequality that exaggerates the $CO_2$ retention. This factor is probably less important than the depression of ventilation, but the rapidity of the rise in arterial $P_{CO_2}$ when some of these patients are given oxygen suggests that this mechanism may play a part.

Such patients present a therapeutic dilemma. On the one hand, oxygen administration is likely to cause severe $CO_2$ retention and respiratory acidosis. On the other hand, it is clearly essential to give some oxygen to relieve the life-threatening hypoxemia. The answer to this problem is to give a relatively low concentration (24–28% $O_2$) and to monitor the arterial blood gases frequently to determine whether depression of ventilation is occurring. Intubation and mechanical ventilation may become necessary. The use of added oxygen is discussed further in Chapter 9.

## *Effects*

Raised levels of $P_{CO_2}$ in the blood greatly increase cerebral blood flow, causing headache, raised CSF pressure, and sometimes, papilledema. In practice, the cerebral effects of hypercapnia overlap with the effects of hypoxemia. The resulting abnormalities include restlessness, tremor, slurred speech, asterixis (flapping tremor), and fluctuations of mood. High levels of $P_{CO_2}$ are narcotic and cloud consciousness.

## Acidosis in Respiratory Failure

The $CO_2$ retention causes a respiratory acidosis that may be severe, especially after the injudicious administration of oxygen. However, patients who gradually develop respiratory failure may retain considerable amounts of bicarbonate, keeping the fall of pH in check (see Figure 2-10).

Metabolic acidosis frequently coexists with respiratory acidosis and complicates the acid–base abnormality. This is caused by the liberation of lactic acid from hypoxic tissues, and the dual factors of hypoxemia and an inadequate peripheral circulation are additive. In patients who are mechanically ventilated, the raised intrathoracic pressure may interfere with venous return and cardiac output and thus further reduce peripheral blood flow.

## Role of Diaphragm Fatigue

Fatigue of the diaphragm can contribute to the hypoventilation of respiratory failure. The diaphragm consists of striated skeletal muscle innervated by the phrenic nerves. Although the diaphragm is predominantly made up of slow-twitch oxidative fibers and fast-twitch oxidative glycolytic fibers, which are relatively resistant to fatigue, this can occur if the work of breathing is greatly increased over prolonged periods of time. Fatigue can be defined as a loss of contractile force after work; it can be measured directly from the transdiaphragmatic pressure resulting from a maximum contraction or indirectly from the muscle relaxation time or the electromyogram. There is evidence that some patients with severe COPD continually breathe close to the work level at which fatigue occurs, and that an exacerbation of infection can tip them into a fatigue state. This will then result in hypoventilation, $CO_2$ retention, and severe hypoxemia. Because hypercapnia impairs diaphragm contractility and severe hypoxemia accelerates the onset of fatigue, a vicious cycle develops.

The dangers of diaphragm fatigue can be limited by reducing the work of breathing by treating bronchospasm and controlling infection, and by giving oxygen judiciously to relieve the hypoxemia. The force of contraction can be improved by a training program, for example, by breathing through inspiratory resistances. In addition, the administration of methylxanthines improves diaphragm contractility and also relieves reversible bronchoconstriction. However, the role of fatigue of the diaphragm in respiratory failure is still not fully understood.

## ▶ Types of Respiratory Failure

A large number of conditions can lead to respiratory failure, and various classifications are possible. However, from the point of view of the physiological principles of management, five groups can be distinguished:

1. Acute overwhelming lung disease

2. Neuromuscular disorders

3. Acute on chronic lung disease

4. ARDS

5. Infant respiratory distress syndrome

## Acute Overwhelming Lung Disease

Many acute diseases, if severe enough, can lead to respiratory failure. These include infections such as fulminating viral or bacterial pneumonias, vascular diseases such as pulmonary embolism, and exposure to inhaled toxic substances such as chlorine gas or oxides of nitrogen. Respiratory failure supervenes as the primary disease progresses, and profound hypoxemia with or without hypercapnia develops. Oxygen administration is required for the hypoxemia, and mechanical ventilation may be necessary to tide the patient over the worst stage. A few patients have been treated by extracorporeal membrane oxygenators that largely take over the gas exchange function of the lung. Treatment of the underlying disease, for example, antibiotics for bacterial pneumonias, is clearly necessary. This group of conditions merges into ARDS (see the section "Adult Respiratory Distress Syndrome" later in this chapter).

## Neuromuscular Disorders

Respiratory failure may occur when the respiratory center is depressed by drugs such as heroin and barbiturates. Other conditions include central nervous system and neuromuscular diseases such as encephalitis, poliomyelitis, Guillain-Barré syndrome, myasthenia gravis, anti-cholinesterase poisoning, amyotrophic lateral sclerosis, and progressive muscular dystrophy (see Figure 2-3 and Table 2-1). Trauma to the chest wall can also be responsible.

In these conditions, the essential feature is hypoventilation leading to $CO_2$ retention with moderate hypoxemia (see Figures 2-2 and 8-1). Respiratory acidosis occurs, but the magnitude of the fall in pH depends on the rapidity of the increase in $P_{CO_2}$ and the extent of the renal compensation.

Mechanical ventilation is often necessary in these conditions and occasionally, as in bulbar poliomyelitis, it may be required for months or even years. However, the lung itself is often normal and, if so, no additional oxygen is necessary to reverse the hypoxemia. Again, treatment of the underlying disease is always indicated, if available.

## Acute on Chronic Lung Disease

This refers to an acute exacerbation of disease in a patient with long-standing underlying disease. It is an important and common group that includes patients with chronic bronchitis and emphysema, asthma, and cystic fibrosis. Many patients with COPD follow a gradual downhill course with increasingly severe hypoxemia and $CO_2$ retention over months or years. Such patients are usually capable of limited physical activity even though both the arterial $P_{O_2}$ and $P_{CO_2}$ may be in the region of 50 mm Hg. As a result, this situation is not conventionally referred to as respiratory failure.

However, if such a patient develops even a mild exacerbation of the chest infection, the condition often deteriorates rapidly, with profound hypoxemia, $CO_2$ retention, and respiratory acidosis. The reserves of pulmonary function are minimal, and any increase in the work of breathing or worsening of ventilation–perfusion relationships as a result of retained secretions or bronchospasm pushes the patient over the brink into frank respiratory failure.

The treatment of these patients requires a delicate touch. Naturally, the underlying infection should be treated with antibiotics. In addition, bronchodilators are indicated for bronchospasm, and diuretics and digitalis may be required if there is evidence of heart failure. Supplemental oxygen is necessary to relieve the severe hypoxemia. However, these patients frequently lose their ventilatory drive and develop severe $CO_2$ retention and acidosis if too much oxygen is administered. For this reason, it is usual to begin with 24-28% oxygen and monitor the arterial blood gases frequently (see Chapter 9).

Mechanical ventilation may be necessary, but the decision on whether to employ this is often difficult. On the one hand, it may be impossible to prevent the rise of arterial $P_{CO_2}$ without assisted ventilation. On the other hand, these patients often have such diseased lungs that once they are on the ventilator, it may be difficult or impossible to wean them from it. Each case must be considered on its merits, but mechanical ventilation should generally be used only if there is a substantial reversible component to the patient's condition.

## Adult Respiratory Distress Syndrome

This condition is sometimes referred to as acute respiratory failure. It is an end result of a variety of insults, including trauma to the lung or to the rest of the body, aspiration, sepsis (especially that caused by gram-negative organisms), and shock from any cause. There is evidence that many other organs are also affected, and the condition should probably be regarded as multiorgan failure.

## Pathology

The early changes consist of interstitial and alveolar edema. Hemorrhage, cellular debris, and proteinaceous fluid are present in the alveoli, hyaline membranes may be seen, and there is patchy atelectasis (Figure 8-2). Later, hyperplasia and organization occur. The damaged alveolar epithelium becomes lined with type 2 alveolar epithelial cells, and there is cellular infiltration of the alveolar walls. Eventually, interstitial fibrosis may develop, although complete healing can occur.

## Pathogenesis

This is still unclear and many factors may play a role. The capillary endothelial and type 1 alveolar epithelial cells are damaged early, causing increased capillary permeability and flooding of the alveoli with proteinaceous fluid. Neutrophils accumulate partly as a result of complement or kinin activation. The activated neutrophils release mediators, including bradykinin, histamine, and platelet activating factor (PAF). In addition, toxic oxygen radicals are generated, together with cyclooxygenase products such as prostaglandins and thromboxane, and also lipoxygenase products such as leukotrienes. Platelets activated by PAF release proteases and kallikrein.

## Clinical Features

ARDS is often associated with some severe underlying medical or surgical illness unconnected with the lung, and the onset of respiratory failure is often delayed. A typical history is that the patient is exposed to severe trauma, for example, an automobile accident with

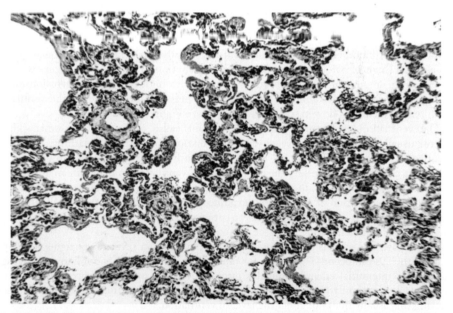

**Figure 8-2.** **Histologic Changes in ARDS as Found by an Open Lung Biopsy.** There are patchy atelectasis, edema, hyaline membranes, and cellular debris in the alveoli. (From Lamy M, Fallat RJ, Koeniger E, et al. Pathologic features and mechanisms of hypoxemia in adult respiratory distress syndrome. *Am Rev Resp Dis* 1976;114:267–284.)

multiple fractures. There is some hemorrhagic shock with hypotension, which is treated by fluid replacement. The patient appears to be doing well when, perhaps 2 days after the trauma, some increase in respiratory rate is noted, the arterial $P_{O_2}$ and $P_{CO_2}$ fall, and clouding is seen in the chest radiograph, which progresses to dense uneven opacification. Severe hypoxemia develops. The mortality rate is high.

## Pulmonary Function

The lung becomes very stiff, and unusually high pressures are required to ventilate it mechanically. Associated with this reduced compliance is a marked fall in FRC. The cause of the increased recoil is presumably the alveolar edema and exudate that exaggerate the surface tension forces. As was pointed out in Chapter 6 (see Figure 6-3), edematous alveoli have a reduced volume. It is also possible that interstitial edema contributes to the abnormal stiffness of the lungs.

### Adult Respiratory Distress Syndrome (ARDS)

End-result of a variety of insults including trauma and infection

Hemorrhagic edema with opacification on the radiograph

Severe hypoxemia

Low lung compliance

Mechanical ventilation typically required

High mortality

As would be expected from the histologic appearance of the lung (Figure 8-2), there is marked ventilation–perfusion inequality, with a substantial fraction of the total blood flow going to unventilated alveoli. This fraction may reach 50% or more. Figure 8-3 shows some results obtained by the multiple inert gas method in a 44-year-old patient who developed respiratory failure after an automobile accident and who was mechanically ventilated. Note the presence of blood flow to lung units with abnormally low ventilation–perfusion ratios and also the shunt of 8% (compare the normal distribution in Figure 2-9). Figure 8-3 also shows a large amount of ventilation going to units with high ventilation–perfusion ratios. One reason for this is the abnormally high airway pressures developed by the ventilator, which reduce the blood flow in some alveoli (compare Figure 10-4).

The ventilation–perfusion inequality and shunt cause profound hypoxemia. These patients usually must be given oxygen-enriched mixtures because air breathing, even with a ventilator, results in an arterial $P_{O_2}$ that is dangerously low. Oxygen concentrations of 40 to 100% are sometimes necessary during mechanical ventilation to maintain an arterial $P_{O_2}$ above 60 mm Hg. However, the possibility of oxygen toxicity should be kept in mind (see Chapter 9). The addition of positive end-expiratory pressure (PEEP) often results in a substantial improvement in oxygenation in these patients (compare Figure 10-4). However high levels of PEEP can damage the lung (see Chapter 10).

By contrast, the arterial $P_{CO_2}$ is sometimes low, even when severe hypoxemia develops; values in the 20s can occur. The reason for the increased ventilation is not known, although possibly the interstitial edema stimulates intrapulmonary J or stretch receptors. Another possible factor is stimulation of the peripheral chemoreceptors by the hypoxemia, although relieving this usually does not affect the level of ventilation.

## Infant Respiratory Distress Syndrome

This condition, which is also called hyaline membrane disease of the newborn, has several features in common with ARDS. Pathologically, the lung shows hemorrhagic edema, patchy atelectasis, and hyaline membranes caused by proteinaceous fluid and cellular debris within the alveoli. Physiologically, there is profound hypoxemia, with both ventilation–perfusion inequality and blood flow through unventilated lung. In addition, a right-to-left shunt via the patent foramen ovale may exaggerate the hypoxemia. Mechanical ventilation with enriched oxygen mixtures is often necessary, and the addition of PEEP or continuous positive air way pressure (see Chapter 10) is frequently beneficial. However these infants may go on to develop bronchopulmonary dysplasia.

The chief cause of this condition is an absence of pulmonary surfactant, although other factors are also probably involved. The surfactant is normally produced by the type 2 alveolar epithelial cells (see Figure 5-2), and the ability of the lung to synthesize adequate amounts of the material develops relatively late in fetal life. Thus, a prematurely born infant is particularly at risk. The ability of the infant to secrete surfactant can be estimated by measuring the lecithin/sphingomyelin ratio of amniotic fluid, and maturation of the surfactant-synthesizing system can be hastened by the administration of corticosteroids. Treatment of the condition by administering exogenous surfactant via the trachea has been a major advance.

## ▶ Management of Respiratory Failure

Although many factors might contribute to the respiratory failure of an individual patient, it is useful to discuss the physiologic principles that underlie a treatment. Naturally, attention must be directed to the primary cause of the disease. For example, antibiotic therapy may be required for an infection, or a specific treatment may be available for a neuromuscular disorder. However, some aspects are common to many patients with respiratory failure.

### Airway Obstruction

Respiratory failure is often precipitated by an increase in airway resistance. Many patients have COPD of many years' duration with hypoxemia and even some mild hypercapnia. Even so, they are able to maintain some physical activity. However, if they develop bronchospasm

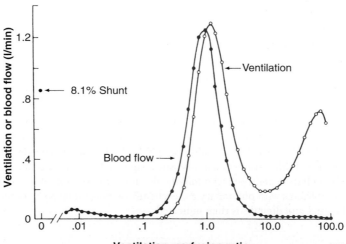

**Figure 9-3.** Distribution of Ventilation–Perfusion Ratios in a Patient Who Developed ARDS **After an Automobile Accident**. Note the 8% shunt and the blood flow to units with low ventilation–perfusion ratios. In addition, there is some ventilation to high $\dot{V}_A/\dot{Q}$ units, probably as a result of the high airway pressure developed by the ventilator (compare Figure 10-4).

through exposure to smog or cold air or if they have a "chesty cold" with an increase in secretions, they may rapidly develop respiratory failure. The additional work of breathing becomes the straw that breaks the camel's back, and they develop profound hypoxemia, $CO_2$ retention, and respiratory acidosis.

Treatment should be directed at reducing the airway obstruction. Retained secretions are best removed by coughing when this is effective. Encouragement to cough and assistance by a respiratory therapist, nurse, or physician is often helpful, and changing the patient's position from side to side to assist drainage of secretions may be beneficial. Adequate hydration is important to prevent the secretions from becoming too viscid. It is especially important to humidify all gases given by a ventilator to prevent thickening and crusting of secretions. Drugs such as potassium iodide by mouth or acetylcysteine by aerosol to liquefy sputum are of doubtful value. Chest physiotherapy may help to clear airway secretions. However, aspiration of secretions by bronchoscopy may become necessary. Occasionally, respiratory stimulants are given to a drowsy patient but, more important, respiratory depressants must be avoided because they suppress coughing.

Any reversible airway obstruction should be treated by bronchodilators, such as albuterol or metaproterenol aerosol, intravenous aminophylline, or perhaps intravenous corticosteroids. Drugs such as isoproterenol that also stimulate $\beta_1$-adrenergic receptors in the heart should be avoided.

## Respiratory Infection

An exacerbation of bronchitis in a patient with COPD, or a fresh respiratory infection in a patient with advanced interstitial lung disease, frequently provokes respiratory failure. There are at least two physiologic mechanisms for this. First, the increased secretions and, perhaps, bronchospasm increase the work of breathing, as discussed earlier. Second, there is a worsening of ventilation–perfusion relationships so that even if the ventilation to the alveoli remains unchanged, there will be increasing hypoxemia and hypercapnia. Vigorous treatment of the infection by antibiotics is indicated.

Even a mild exacerbation of bronchitis in a patient with COPD may precipitate respiratory failure. Moreover, the usual systemic responses to infection, such as pyrexia and leukocytosis, are often absent. However, treatment should not be delayed.

## Cardiac Insufficiency

Many patients with incipient respiratory failure have a compromised cardiovascular system. The pulmonary artery pressure is frequently raised as a result of several factors, including destruction of the pulmonary capillary bed by disease, hypoxic vasoconstriction, and perhaps increased blood viscosity caused by polycythemia. In addition, the myocardium is chronically hypoxic. Fluid retention often occurs as a result of retention of bicarbonate and sodium ions by the hypoxic kidney. Finally, some patients have coexisting coronary artery disease.

Patients with COPD frequently develop peripheral edema, hepatomegaly, and engorged neck veins. These and other patients may also show signs of left heart failure, with basal rales (crackles) on auscultation and engorged lung fields on the radiograph. The mild pulmonary edema further interferes with pulmonary gas exchange by causing uneven ventilation. Treatment with diuretics and digitalis is then indicated.

## Hypoxemia

Hypoxemia can be relieved to some extent by treating the airway obstruction and the chest infection. However, the administration of long-term oxygen is frequently required, and this important topic is discussed in detail in Chapter 9.

# Hypercapnia

Hypercapnia often responds to general measures directed at the airway obstruction and the infection. However, mechanical ventilation is frequently required. This is discussed in detail in Chapter 10.

## KEY CONCEPTS

1. Respiratory failure refers to the condition when the lung fails to oxygenate the blood adequately or fails to prevent $CO_2$ retention.

2. The four causes of hypoxemia are hyperventilation, diffusion impairment, shunt, and ventilation–perfusion inequality, and the causes of $CO_2$ retention are hypoventilation and ventilation-perfusion inequality.

3. Severe hypoxemia causes many abnormalities including mental confusion, tachycardia, lactic acidemia, and proteinuria. $CO_2$ retention increases cerebral blood flow and may result in headache and confusion.

4. Gas exchange abnormalities in respiratory failure vary depending on the causative disease. For example, the ARDS is characterized by severe hypoxemia with or without $CO_2$ retention. However, in pure hypoventilation, as in neuromuscular disease, $CO_2$ retention and respiratory acidosis dominate.

5. Management of respiratory failure may include relieving airway obstruction, treating infection, and administering oxygen, and in some cases instituting mechanical ventilation.

## QUESTIONS

1. A patient was admitted to the hospital with an acute pulmonary exacerbation of chronic pulmonary disease. When given 100% oxygen to breathe, his arterial $P_{CO_2}$ increased from 50 to 80 mm Hg. A likely cause was:
   A. Increased airway resistance.
   B. Depression of ventilation.
   C. Depression of cardiac output.
   D. Reduced levels of 2,3-diphosphoglycerate in the blood.
   E. Bohr effect.

2. Respiratory acidosis in respiratory failure is likely to be increased by:
   A. Mechanical ventilation.
   B. Exacerbation of a chest infection.
   C. Treatment with digitalis.
   D. Renal retention of bicarbonate.
   E. Administration of antibiotics.

3. The Adult Respiratory Distress Syndrome (ARDS) is likely to include:
   A. Increased lung compliance.
   B. Increased FRC.
   C. Negligible shunt.
   D. Severe hypoxemia.
   E. Normal chest radiograph.

**4.** A feature of the infant respiratory distress syndrome is:

    A. Excessive formation of pulmonary surfactant.

    B. Patchy hemorrhagic edema and atelectasis in the lung.

    C. Normal arterial $P_{O_2}$.

    D. Small shunt.

    E. Increased incidence after an unusually long gestation.

**5.** An acute exacerbation of bronchitis in a patient with advanced COPD typically results in:

    A. Reduced work of breathing.

    B. Worsening of ventilation–perfusion relationships.

    C. Increased arterial pH.

    D. Reduced alveolar–arterial $P_{O_2}$ difference.

    E. Immediate requirement for mechanical ventilation.

# Oxygen Therapy

# 9

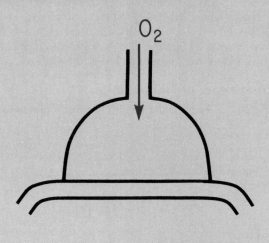

O xygen administration has a critical role in the treatment of hypoxemia and especially in the management of respiratory failure. However, patients vary considerably in their response to oxygen, and several potential hazards are associated with its use. A clear understanding of the physiologic principles involved is necessary to prevent abuses of this powerful agent.

## ▶  Improved Oxygenation After Oxygen Administration

### Power of Added Oxygen

The great extent to which the arterial $P_{O_2}$ can be increased by the inhalation of 100% oxygen is sometimes not appreciated. Suppose a young man has taken an overdose of a narcotic drug that results in severe hypoventilation with an arterial $P_{O_2}$ of 50 mm Hg and a $P_{CO_2}$ of 80 mm Hg (see Figure 2-2). If this patient is mechanically ventilated and given 100% oxygen, the arterial $P_{O_2}$ may increase to over 600 mm Hg, that is, a 10-fold increase (Figure 9-1). Few drugs can improve the gas composition of the blood so greatly and so effortlessly!

### Response of Various Types of Hypoxemia

The mechanism of hypoxemia has an important bearing on its response to inhaled oxygen.

#### *Hypoventilation*

The rise in alveolar $P_{O_2}$ can be predicted from the alveolar gas equation *if* the ventilation and metabolic rate, and therefore the alveolar $P_{CO_2}$, remain unaltered:

$$P_{A_{O_2}} = P_{I_{O_2}} - \frac{P_{A_{CO_2}}}{R} + F, \qquad \text{(Eq. 9.1)}$$

where F is a small correction factor.

Assuming no change in the alveolar $P_{CO_2}$ and the respiratory exchange ratio, and neglecting the correction factor, this equation shows that the alveolar $P_{O_2}$ rises in parallel with the inspired value. Thus changing from air to only 30% oxygen can increase the alveolar $P_{O_2}$ by approximately 60 mm Hg. In practice, the arterial $P_{O_2}$ is always lower than the alveolar value because of a small amount of venous admixture. However, the hypoxemia of hypoventilation, which is rarely severe (see Figure 2-2), is easily reversed by a modest oxygen enrichment of the inspired gas.

#### *Diffusion Impairment*

Again, hypoxemia caused by this mechanism is readily overcome by oxygen administration. The reason for this becomes clear if we look at the dynamics of oxygen uptake along the

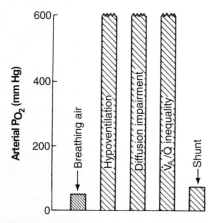

**Figure 9-1. Response of the Arterial $P_{O_2}$ to 100% Inspired Oxygen for Mechanisms of Hypoxemia.** The $P_{O_2}$ breathing air is assumed to be 50 mm Hg. Note the dramatic increase in all instances except shunt where, nevertheless, there is a useful gain.

pulmonary capillary (see Figure 2-4). The rate of movement of oxygen across the blood–gas barrier is proportional to the $P_{O_2}$ difference between alveolar gas and capillary blood. (See *Respiratory Physiology: The Essentials*, 9th ed., p. 30). This difference is normally approximately 60 mm Hg at the beginning of the capillary. If we increase the concentration of inspired oxygen to only 30%, we raise the alveolar $P_{O_2}$ by 60 mm Hg, thus doubling the rate of transfer of oxygen at the start of the capillary. This in turn improves oxygenation of the end-capillary blood. Therefore, a modest rise in inspired oxygen concentration can usually correct the hypoxemia.

### Ventilation–Perfusion Inequality

Again, oxygen administration usually is very effective at improving the arterial $P_{O_2}$. However, the rise in $P_{O_2}$ depends on the pattern of ventilation–perfusion inequality and the inspired oxygen concentration. Administration of 100% $O_2$ increases the arterial $P_{O_2}$ to high values because every lung unit that is ventilated eventually washes out its nitrogen. When this occurs, the alveolar $P_{O_2}$ is given by $P_{O_2} = P_B - P_{H_2O} - P_{CO_2}$. Because the $P_{CO_2}$ is normally less than 50 mm Hg, this equation predicts an alveolar $P_{O_2}$ of over 600 mm Hg, even in lung units with very low ventilation–perfusion ratios.

However, two cautions should be added. First, some regions of the lung may be so poorly ventilated that it may take several minutes for the nitrogen to be washed out. Furthermore, these regions may continue to receive nitrogen as this gas is gradually washed out of peripheral tissues by the venous blood. As a consequence, the arterial $P_{O_2}$ may take so long to reach its final level that, in practice, this is never achieved. Second, giving oxygen may result in the development of unventilated areas (Figure 9-5). If this occurs, the rise in arterial $P_{O_2}$ stops short (Figure 9-3).

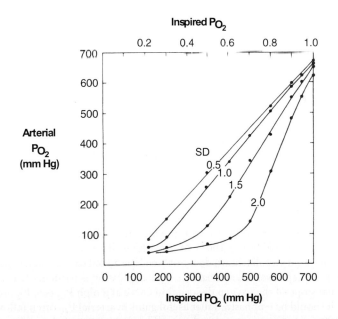

**Figure 9-2. Response of the Arterial $P_{O_2}$ to Various Inspired Oxygen Values in Theoretical Distributions of Ventilation–Perfusion Ratios.** *SD* refers to the standard deviation of the log normal distribution. Note that when the distribution is broad (SD = 2), the arterial $P_{O_2}$ remains low even when 60% oxygen is inhaled. (From West JB, Wagner PD. Pulmonary gas exchange. In: West JB. ed. *Bioengineering Aspects of the Lung*. New York, NY: Marcel Dekker, 1977.)

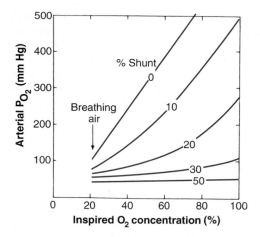

**Figure 9-3. Response of the Arterial P$_{O_2}$ to Increased Inspired Oxygen Concentrations in a Lung with Various Amounts of Shunt.** Note that the P$_{O_2}$ remains far below the normal level for 100% oxygen. Nevertheless, useful gains in oxygenation occur even with severe degrees of shunting. (This diagram shows typical values only; changes in cardiac output, oxygen uptake, etc., affect the position of the lines.)

When intermediate concentrations of oxygen are given, the rise in arterial P$_{O_2}$ is determined by the pattern of ventilation–perfusion inequality and in particular by those units that have low ventilation–perfusion ratios and appreciable blood flow. Figure 9-2 shows the response of the arterial P$_{O_2}$ in lung models with various distributions of ventilation–perfusion ratios after inspiration of various oxygen concentrations. Note that at an inspired concentration of 60%, the arterial P$_{O_2}$ of the distribution with a standard deviation of 2.0 rose from 40 to only 90 mm Hg. This modest rise can be attributed to the effects of lung units with ventilation–perfusion ratios less than 0.01. For example, an alveolus with a ventilation–perfusion ratio of 0.006 that is given 60% O$_2$ to inspire has an end-capillary P$_{O_2}$ of only 60 mm Hg in the example shown. However, note that when the inspired oxygen concentration was increased to 90%, the arterial P$_{O_2}$ of this distribution rose to nearly 500 mm Hg.

Figure 9-2 assumes that the pattern of ventilation–perfusion inequality remains constant as the inspired oxygen is raised. However, the relief of alveolar hypoxia in poorly ventilated regions of the lung may increase the blood flow there because of the abolition of hypoxic vasoconstriction. In this case, the increase in arterial P$_{O_2}$ will be less. Note also that if units with low ventilation–perfusion ratios collapse during high oxygen breathing (Figure 9-5), the arterial P$_{O_2}$ rises less.

### Shunt

This is the only mechanism of hypoxemia in which the arterial P$_{O_2}$ remains far below the level for the normal lung during 100% O$_2$ breathing. The reason is that the blood that bypasses the ventilated alveoli (shunt) does not "see" the added oxygen and, being low in oxygen concentration, depresses the arterial P$_{O_2}$. This depression is particularly marked because of the nearly flat slope of the oxygen dissociation curve at a high P$_{O_2}$ (see Figure 2-6).

However, it should be emphasized that useful gains in arterial P$_{O_2}$ often follow the administration of 100% O$_2$ to patients with shunts. This is because of the additional dissolved oxygen, which can be appreciable at a high alveolar P$_{O_2}$. For example, increasing the alveolar P$_{O_2}$ from 100 to 600 mm Hg raises the dissolved oxygen in the end-capillary blood from 0.3 to 1.8 ml of O$_2$/100 ml of blood. This increase of 1.5 can be compared with the normal arterial–venous difference in oxygen concentration of approximately 5 ml/100 ml.

Figure 9-3 shows typical increases in arterial $P_{O_2}$ for various percentage shunts at different inspired oxygen concentrations. The graph is drawn for an oxygen uptake of 300 ml/min and a cardiac output of 6 liters/min; variations in these and other values alter the positions of the lines. However, in this example, a patient with a 30% shunt who has an arterial $P_{O_2}$ of 55 mm Hg during air breathing increases this to 110 mm Hg if he or she breathes 100% oxygen. This increase corresponds to a rise in oxygen saturation and concentration of the arterial blood of 10% and 2.2 ml/100 ml, respectively. In a patient with a hypoxic myocardium, for example, these values mean an important gain in oxygen delivery.

## Important Factors in Oxygen Delivery to Tissues

- Arterial $P_{O_2}$
- Hemoglobin concentration
- Cardiac output
- Diffusion from capillaries to mitochondria (e.g., number of open capillaries)
- Oxygen affinity of hemoglobin
- Local blood flow

## Other Factors in Oxygen Delivery

Although the arterial $P_{O_2}$ is a convenient measurement of the degree of oxygenation of the blood, other factors are important in oxygen delivery to the tissues. These factors include the hemoglobin concentration, the position of the oxygen dissociation curve, the cardiac output, and the distribution of the blood flow throughout the peripheral tissues.

Both a fall in hemoglobin concentration and cardiac output reduce the amount of oxygen per unit time ("oxygen flux") going to the tissues. The flux may be expressed as the product of the cardiac output and the arterial oxygen concentration: $\dot{Q} \times Ca_{O_2}$.

Diffusion of oxygen from the peripheral capillaries to the mitochondria in the tissue cells depends on capillary $P_{O_2}$. A useful index is the $P_{O_2}$ of mixed venous blood, which reflects the average tissue $P_{O_2}$. A rearrangement of the Fick equation is as follows:

$$C\overline{v}_{O_2} = Ca_{O_2} - \frac{\dot{V}_{O_2}}{\dot{Q}} \qquad \text{(Eq. 9.2)}$$

This equation shows that the oxygen concentration (and therefore the $P_{O_2}$) of mixed venous blood will fall if either the arterial oxygen concentration or the cardiac output is reduced (oxygen consumption is assumed constant).

The relationship between oxygen concentration and $P_{O_2}$ in the mixed venous blood depends on the position of the oxygen dissociation curve (see Figure 2-1). If the curve is shifted to the right by an increase in temperature, as in fever, or an increase in 2,3-diphosphoglycerate (DPG) concentration, as may occur in chronic hypoxemia, the $P_{O_2}$ for a given concentration is high, thus favoring diffusion of oxygen to the mitochondria. By contrast, if the $P_{CO_2}$ is low and the pH is high, as in respiratory alkalosis, or if the 2,3-DPG concentration is low because of transfusion of large amounts of stored blood, the resulting left-shifted curve interferes with oxygen unloading to the tissues.

Finally, the distribution of cardiac output clearly plays an important role in tissue oxygenation. For example, a patient who has coronary artery disease is liable to have hypoxic regions in the myocardium, irrespective of the other factors involved in oxygen delivery.

## ▶ Methods of Oxygen Administration

## Nasal Cannulas

Nasal cannulas consist of two prongs that are inserted just inside the anterior nares and supported on a light frame. Oxygen is supplied at rates of 1 to 4 liters/min, resulting in inspired oxygen concentrations of approximately 25 to 30%. The higher the patient's inspiratory flow rate, the lower the resulting concentration. The gas should be humidified as close to body temperature as possible to prevent crusting of secretions on the nasal mucosa.

The chief advantage of cannulas is that the patient does not have the discomfort of a mask and he or she can talk and eat and has access to the face. The cannulas can be worn continuously for long periods, an important point because oxygen administration should usually be continuous rather than intermittent (see later). The disadvantages of cannulas are the low maximum inspired concentrations of oxygen that are available and the unpredictability of the concentration, especially if the patient breathes mostly through the mouth.

## Masks

Masks come in several designs. Simple plastic masks that fit over the nose and mouth allow inspired oxygen concentrations of up to 60% when supplied with flow rates of 6 liters/min. However, because some accumulation of $CO_2$ occurs within the mask (up to 2%), this device should be used with caution for patients who are liable to develop $CO_2$ retention. In addition, some patients report feeling smothered when this type of mask is used.

A useful mask for delivering controlled oxygen concentrations is based on the Venturi principle. As the oxygen enters the mask through a narrow jet, it entrains a constant flow of air, which enters via surrounding holes. With an oxygen flow of 4 liters/min, a total flow (oxygen + air) of approximately 40 liters/min is delivered to the patient. At such high flow rates, there is negligible rebreathing of expired gas and, therefore, no $CO_2$ accumulation. Masks that give inspired oxygen concentrations of 24, 28, or 35% with a high degree of reliability are available and are particularly useful for treating patients who are liable to develop $CO_2$ retention. Some patients complain of the noise and the breeze, while others enjoy the latter.

## Transtracheal Oxygen

This can be delivered via a microcatheter inserted through the anterior tracheal wall with the tip lying just above the carina. It is an efficient way of delivering oxygen, particularly for patients on long-term oxygen therapy, although care must be taken to prevent infection.

## Tents

These are now used only for children who do not tolerate masks well. Oxygen concentrations of up to 50% can be obtained, but there is a fire hazard.

## Ventilators

When a patient is mechanically ventilated through an endotracheal or tracheostomy tube, complete control over the composition of the inspired gas is available. There is a danger of producing oxygen toxicity if concentrations of over 50% are given for more than 2 days (see later). In general, the lowest inspired oxygen that provides an acceptable arterial $P_{O_2}$ should be used. This level is difficult to define, but in patients with acute respiratory distress syndrome (ARDS) who are being mechanically ventilated with high oxygen concentrations, a figure of 60 mm Hg is often used.

## Hyperbaric Oxygen

If 100% $O_2$ is administered at a pressure of 3 atmospheres, the inspired $P_{O_2}$ is over 2000 mm Hg. Under these conditions, a substantial increase in the arterial oxygen concentration can occur, chiefly as a result of additional dissolved oxygen. For example, if the arterial $P_{O_2}$ is 2000 mm Hg, the oxygen in solution is approximately 6 ml/100 ml of blood. Theoretically, this is enough to provide the entire arterial–venous difference of 5 ml/100 ml, so that the hemoglobin of the mixed venous blood could remain fully saturated.

Hyperbaric oxygen therapy has limited uses and is rarely indicated in the treatment of respiratory failure. However, it has been used in the treatment of severe carbon monoxide poisoning where most of the hemoglobin is unavailable to carry oxygen and therefore the dissolved oxygen is critically important. In addition, the high $P_{O_2}$ accelerates the dissociation of carbon monoxide from hemoglobin. A severe anemic crisis is sometimes treated in the same way. Hyperbaric oxygen is also used in the treatment of gas gangrene infections and as an adjunct to radiotherapy where the higher tissue $P_{O_2}$ increases the radiosensitivity of relatively avascular tumors. The high pressure chamber is also valuable for managing decompression sickness.

The use of hyperbaric oxygen requires a special facility with trained personnel. In practice, the chamber is filled with air, and oxygen is given by a special mask to ensure that the patient receives pure oxygen. This procedure also reduces fire hazard.

## Domiciliary and Portable Oxygen

Some patients are so disabled by severe chronic pulmonary disease that they are virtually confined to bed or a chair unless they breathe supplementary oxygen. These patients often benefit considerably from having a supply of oxygen in their home. This can take various forms. A central large tank with a long plastic tube and mask may enable the patient to climb stairs or go to the bathroom. In addition, portable oxygen sets are available, and these can be used for shopping or other activities. Some sets use liquid oxygen as a store; these are best for patient mobility. In others, oxygen is extracted from the air with a molecular sieve.

The patients who benefit most from portable oxygen are those whose exercise tolerance is limited by dyspnea. Increasing the inspired oxygen concentration can greatly increase the level of exercise for a given ventilation and so enable these patients to become much more active.

It has been shown that a low flow of oxygen given continuously over several months can reduce the amount of pulmonary hypertension and improve the prognosis of some patients with advanced chronic obstructive pulmonary disease (COPD). Although such therapy is expensive, improvements in the technology of providing oxygen have made it feasible.

---

## ▶ Hazards of Oxygen Therapy

### Carbon Dioxide Retention

The reasons for the development of dangerous $CO_2$ retention after oxygen administration to patients with severe COPD were briefly discussed in Chapter 8. A critical factor in the ventilatory drive of these patients who have a high work of breathing is often the hypoxic stimulation of their peripheral chemoreceptors. If this is removed by relieving their hypoxemia, the level of ventilation may fall precipitously and severe $CO_2$ retention may ensue.

Intermittent oxygen therapy is especially dangerous. The physiologist Haldane compared this with bringing a drowning man to the surface—occasionally! The explanation is that if oxygen administration is seen to cause $CO_2$ retention and is therefore stopped, the subsequent hypoxemia may be more severe than it was before oxygen therapy. The reason is the increased alveolar $P_{CO_2}$, as can be seen from the alveolar gas equation:

$$P_{A_{O_2}} = P_{I_{O_2}} - \frac{P_{A_{CO_2}}}{R} + F,$$  (Eq. 9.3)

This shows that any increase in alveolar $P_{CO_2}$ will reduce the alveolar $P_{O_2}$ and therefore the arterial value. Moreover, the high $P_{CO_2}$ is likely to remain for many minutes because the body stores of this gas are so great that the excess is wa shed out only gradually. Thus, the hypoxemia may be severe and prolonged.

These patients should be given continuous oxygen at a low concentration, and the blood gases must be monitored. Initially, an oxygen concentration of 24% is often given by means of a Venturi mask, and the arterial $P_{O_2}$ and $P_{CO_2}$ are measured after 15 to 20 minutes. If the $P_{CO_2}$ does not rise more than a few mm Hg and the patient remains alert, the oxygen concentration can be increased to 28%. This is generally adequate to relieve severe hypoxemia, although concentrations as high as 35% are sometimes used. The shape of the oxygen dissociation curve (see Figure 2-1) should be at the back of the physician's mind to remind him or her that a rise in $P_{O_2}$ from 30 to 50 mm Hg (at a normal pH) represents more than a 25% increase in hemoglobin saturation!

## Oxygen Toxicity

High concentrations of oxygen over long periods damage the lung. Studies of monkeys exposed to 100% oxygen for 2 days show that some of the earliest changes are in the capillary endothelial cells, which become swollen. Alterations occur in the endothelial intercellular junctions, and there is an increased capillary permeability that leads to interstitial and alveolar edema. In addition, the alveolar epithelium may become denuded and replaced by rows of type 2 epithelial cells. Later, organization occurs with interstitial fibrosis.

In humans, the pulmonary effects of high oxygen concentration are more difficult to document, but normal subjects report substernal discomfort after breathing 100% oxygen for 24 hours. Patients who have been mechanically ventilated with 100% oxygen for 36 hours have shown a progressive fall in arterial $P_{O_2}$ compared with a control group who were ventilated with air. A reasonable attitude is to assume that oxygen concentrations of 50% or higher for more than 2 days may produce toxic changes.

In practice, such high levels over such a long period can be achieved only in patients who are intubated and mechanically ventilated. It is important to avoid oxygen toxicity because the only way to relieve the resultant hypoxemia is by raising the inspired oxygen, thus creating a vicious cycle.

## Atelectasis

### Following Airway Occlusion

If a patient is breathing air and an airway becomes totally obstructed, for example, by retained secretions, absorption atelectasis of the lung behind the airway may occur. The reason is that the sum of the partial pressures in the venous blood is considerably less than atmospheric pressure, with the result that the trapped gas is gradually absorbed. (See *Respiratory Physiology: The Essentials*, 9th ed., p. 155.) However, the process is relatively slow, requiring many hours or even days.

However, if the patient is breathing a high concentration of oxygen, the rate of absorption atelectasis is greatly accelerated. This is because there is then relatively little nitrogen in the alveoli and this gas normally slows the absorption process because of its low solubility.

Replacing the nitrogen with any other gas that is rapidly absorbed also predisposes to collapse. An example is nitrous oxide during anesthesia. In the normal lung, collateral ventilation may delay or prevent atelectasis by providing an alternative path for gas to enter the obstructed region (see Figure 1-11C).

Absorption atelectasis is common in patients with respiratory failure because they often have excessive secretions or cellular debris in their airways and they are frequently treated with high oxygen concentrations. In addition, the channels through which collateral ventilation normally occurs may be obstructed by disease. Collapse is common in the dependent regions of the lung because secretions tend to collect there, and those airways and alveoli are relatively poorly expanded anyway (see Figure 3-5). Hypoxemia develops to the extent that atelectatic lung is perfused, although hypoxic vasoconstriction may limit this to some extent.

## Instability of Units with Low Ventilation–Perfusion Ratios

It has been shown that lung units with low ventilation–perfusion ratios may become unstable and collapse when high oxygen mixtures are inhaled. An example is given in Figure 9-4, which shows the distribution of ventilation–perfusion ratios in a patient during air breathing and after 30 minutes of 100% oxygen. This patient had respiratory failure after an automobile accident (see Figure 8-3). Note that during air breathing there were appreciable amounts of blood flow to lung units with low ventilation–perfusion ratios in addition to an 8% shunt. After oxygen administration, the blood flow to the low ventilation–perfusion ratio units was not evident, but the shunt had increased to nearly 16%. The most likely explanation of this change is that the poorly ventilated regions became unventilated.

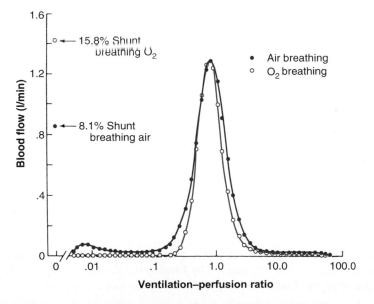

**Figure 9-4. Conversion of Low Ventilation–Perfusion Ratio Units to Shunt During Oxygen Breathing.** This patient had respiratory failure after an automobile accident (same patient as shown in Figure 8-3). During air breathing there was appreciable blood flow to units with low ventilation–perfusion ratios. After 30 minutes of 100% oxygen, blood flow to these units was not evident, but the shunt doubled.

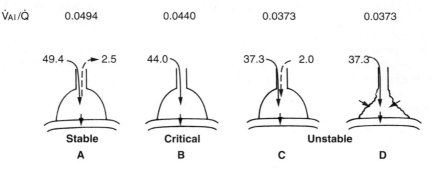

Inspired $O_2$ = 80%

$\dot{V}_{AI}/\dot{Q}$     0.0494          0.0440          0.0373          0.0373

49.4  →  2.5       44.0          37.3  →  2.0       37.3

Stable          Critical                Unstable
A                 B                 C                 D

**Figure 9-5.** Mechanism of the Collapse of Lung Units with Low Inspired Ventilation–Perfusion Ratios ($\dot{V}_{AI}/\dot{Q}$) When High Oxygen Mixtures Are Inhaled. **A.** The expired ventilation is very small because so much of the inspired gas is taken up by the blood. **C,D.** More gas is removed from the lung unit than is inspired, leading to an unstable condition.

Figure 9-5 shows the mechanism involved. The figure shows four hypothetical lung units, all with low inspired ventilation–perfusion ratios ( $V_A/\dot{Q}$ ) during 80% oxygen breathing. In A, the inspired (alveolar) ventilation is 49.4 units but the expired ventilation is only 2.5 units (the actual values depend on the blood flow). The reason why so little gas is exhaled is that so much is taken up by the blood. In B, where the inspired ventilation is slightly reduced to 44.0 units (same blood flow as before), there is no expired ventilation because all the gas that is inspired is absorbed by the blood. Such a unit is said to have a "critical" ventilation–perfusion ratio.

In Figure 9-5C and D, the inspired ventilation has been further reduced with the result that it is now less than the volume of gas entering the blood. This is an unstable situation. Under these circumstances, either gas is inspired from neighboring units during the expiratory phase of respiration, as in C, or the unit gradually collapses, as in D. The latter fate is particularly likely if the unit is poorly ventilated because of intermittent airway closure. This is probably common in the dependent regions of the lung in ARDS because of the greatly reduced FRC. The likelihood of atelectasis increases rapidly as the inspired oxygen concentration approaches 100%.

The development of shunts during oxygen breathing is an additional reason to avoid, if possible, high concentrations of this gas in the treatment of patients with respiratory failure. Also, the shunt that is measured during 100% oxygen breathing (see Figure 2-6) in these patients may substantially overestimate the shunt that is present during air breathing.

## Retrolental Fibroplasia

If newborn infants with the infant respiratory distress syndrome are treated with high concentrations of oxygen, they may develop fibrosis behind the lens of the eye, leading to blindness. This has been successfully avoided by keeping the arterial $P_{O_2}$ below 140 mm Hg. Recently, however, the disease has reappeared for reasons that are not clear.

## KEY CONCEPTS

1. Oxygen therapy is extremely valuable in the treatment of many patients with lung disease, and it can often greatly increase the arterial $P_{O_2}$.

2. The response of the arterial $P_{O_2}$ to inhaled oxygen varies considerably depending on the cause of the hypoxemia. Patients with large shunts do not respond well, although even here the increase in arterial $P_{O_2}$ can be helpful.

3. Various methods of oxygen administration are available. Nasal cannulas are valuable for long-term treatment of patients with COPD. The highest inspired oxygen concentrations are obtained with intubation and mechanical ventilation.

4. Hazards of oxygen therapy include oxygen toxicity, carbon dioxide retention, carbon dioxide retention, atelectasis, and retrolental fibroplasia.

## QUESTIONS

1. A previously well young man was admitted to the emergency department with acute barbiturate poisoning that caused severe hypoventilation. When he was given 50% oxygen to breathe, there was no change in his arterial $P_{CO_2}$. Approximately how much would his arterial $P_{O_2}$ (mm Hg) be expected to rise?

   A. 25
   B. 50
   C. 75
   D. 100
   E. 200

2. A patient with congenital heart disease has a right-to-left shunt and an arterial $P_{O_2}$ of 60 mm Hg during air breathing. When he is given 100% oxygen to breathe, you would expect his arterial $P_{O_2}$ to:

   A. Fall.
   B. Remain unchanged.
   C. Increase by less than 10 mm Hg.
   D. Increase by more than 10 mm Hg.
   E. Rise to about 600 mm Hg.

3. A blood sample from a patient with carbon monoxide poisoning showed a reduction in $P_{50}$ of the oxygen dissociation curve. The probable reason was:

   A. Increased arterial $P_{O_2}$.
   B. The presence of carbon monoxide increased the oxygen affinity of the hemoglobin.
   C. The concentration of 2,3-DPG in the red cells was increased.
   D. Reduced arterial pH.
   E. Mild pyrexia.

4. A disadvantage of nasal cannulas for oxygen administration compared with masks is:

   A. They are more uncomfortable than masks.
   B. Inspired oxygen concentrations above 25% are impossible to obtain.
   C. The inspired oxygen concentration varies considerably.
   D. The patient cannot talk.
   E. The inspired $P_{CO_2}$ tends to rise.

5. A patient with normal lungs but severe anemia is placed in a hyperbaric chamber, total pressure 3 atmospheres, and 100% oxygen is administered by valve box. You can expect the dissolved oxygen in the arterial blood (in ml $O_2$/100 ml blood) to increase to:

   A. 1
   B. 2
   C. 3
   D. 4
   E. 6

6. If 100% oxygen is delivered to the lung over a long period of time, histologic changes of oxygen toxicity occur. The first changes are probably in the:

   A. Type 1 alveolar epithelial cells.
   B. Type 2 alveolar epithelial cells.
   C. Interstitial cells.
   D. Capillary endothelial cells.
   E. Alveolar macrophages.

7. Lung units with low ventilation–perfusion ratios may collapse when high concentrations of oxygen are inhaled for 1 hour, because:

   A. Pulmonary surfactant is inactivated.
   B. Oxygen toxicity causes alveolar edema.
   C. Gas is taken up by the blood faster than it can enter the units by ventilation.
   D. Interstitial edema around the small airways causes airway closure.
   E. Inflammatory changes occur in the small airways.

# Mechanical Ventilation

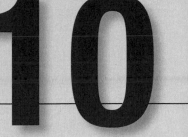

**10**

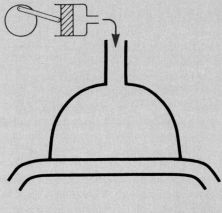

Mechanical ventilation is of major importance in treating patients with respiratory failure. Once used only as an emergency procedure in resuscitation or as a last resort in the treatment of the critically ill, it is now frequently employed to tide a patient over a respiratory crisis. Mechanical ventilation is a complex and technical subject, and this discussion is limited to the physiologic principles of its use, benefits, and hazards.

## ▶ Intubation and Tracheostomy

Most ventilators require a port for connection to the lung airway. An exception is the tank type of ventilator (see later in this chapter), which is now rarely used. The connection is made by means of an endotracheal or, less commonly, a tracheostomy tube. These tubes are provided with an inflatable cuff at the end to give an airtight seal. Endotracheal tubes can be inserted via the nose or mouth.

These tubes have additional functions besides providing a connection for ventilators. They facilitate the removal of secretions by suction catheter, a serious problem in many patients with respiratory failure. Retained secretions are particularly troublesome in patients who are obtunded, who have a suppressed cough reflex, or in whom the secretions are particularly copious or viscid. In addition, a tracheostomy may be necessary to bypass upper airway obstruction caused, for example, by allergic edema or a laryngeal tumor. The tube may also prevent the aspiration of blood or vomitus from the pharynx into the lung.

The decision to intubate and ventilate a patient should not be lightly undertaken because it is a major intervention that requires a substantial investment of personnel and equipment, with many hazards. However, patients are frequently intubated too late in the course of respiratory failure. The precise timing depends on such factors as the nature of the underlying disease process, the rapidity of the progress of hypoxemia and hypercapnia, and the age and general condition of the patient.

Several complications are associated with endotracheal and tracheostomy tubes. Ulceration of the larynx or the trachea is sometimes seen. This complication is particularly likely if the inflated cuff exerts undue pressure on the mucosa; furthermore, the subsequent scarring can result in tracheal stenosis. The use of large-volume, low-pressure cuffs has reduced the incidence of this problem. Also, care must be taken with the placement of an endotracheal tube. For example, if the distal end of the tube is inadvertently placed in the right main bronchus, atelectasis of the left lung may ensue.

## ▶ Types of Ventilators

### Constant-Volume Ventilators

These ventilators deliver a preset volume of gas to the patient, usually by means of a motor-driven piston in a cylinder (Figure 10-1) or a motor-driven bellows. The stroke and frequency of the pump can be adjusted to give the required ventilation. The ratio of inspiratory to expiratory time can also be controlled by a special switching mechanism. Oxygen can be added to the inspired air as required, and a humidifier is included in the circuit.

Constant-volume ventilators are robust, dependable machines that are suitable for long-term ventilation. They are used extensively in anesthesia. They have the advantage of having a known volume (or nearly so) delivered to the patient despite changes in the elastic properties of the lung or chest wall or increases in airway resistance. A disadvantage is that high pressures can be developed; however, in practice, a safety blow-off valve prevents pressures from reaching dangerous levels. Estimating the patient's ventilation from the stroke volume and frequency of the pump may lead to important errors because of the compressibility of the gas and leaks, and it is better to measure the expired ventilation with a spirometer.

### Constant-Pressure Ventilators

These ventilators deliver gas at a preset pressure and are small, relatively inexpensive machines. They do not require electrical power but instead work off a source of compressed gas having a pressure of at least 50 pounds per square inch. Their chief disadvantage, if they

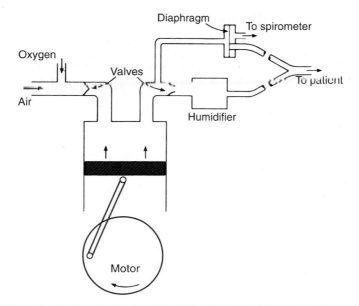

**Figure 10-1. Example of a Constant-Volume Ventilator (Schematic).** In practice, the stroke volume and frequency can be regulated. During the expiratory phase, as the piston descends, the diaphragm is deflected to the left by the reduced pressure in the cylinder, allowing the patient to exhale through the spirometer.

are used as the sole method of ventilation, is that the volume of gas they deliver is altered by changes in the compliance of the lung or chest wall. Also, an increase in airway resistance may decrease the ventilation because there may be insufficient time for equilibration of pressure between the machine and the alveoli. Expired volume should, therefore, be monitored. This is difficult with some ventilators. Another disadvantage of some constant-pressure ventilators is that the inspired oxygen concentration varies with the inspiratory flow rate.

Constant-pressure ventilators are now mainly used for "pressure-assist ventilation," that is, to assist intubated patients to overcome the increased work of breathing occasioned by the relatively narrow endotracheal tube. This mode of use is valuable in weaning patients from a ventilator, that is, in the transition from mechanical ventilation to spontaneous ventilation.

## Tank Ventilators

The ventilators we have discussed up to this point are called positive pressure ventilators because they expand the lung by delivering positive pressure to the airway. By contrast, tank respirators deliver negative pressure (less than atmospheric) to the outside of the chest and rest of the body, excluding the head. They consist of a rigid box (iron lung) connected to a large-volume, low-pressure pump that controls the respiratory cycle. The box is often hinged along the middle so that it can be opened to allow nursing care.

Tank ventilators are no longer used in the treatment of acute respiratory failure because they limit access to the patient and because they are bulky and inconvenient. They were employed extensively to ventilate patients with bulbar poliomyelitis, and they are still occasionally useful for patients with chronic neuromuscular disease who need to be ventilated for months or years. A modification of the tank ventilator is the cuirass, which fits over the thorax and abdomen and also generates negative pressure. It is usually reserved for patients who have partially recovered from neuromuscular respiratory failure.

## Patient-Cycled Ventilators

In these ventilators, the inspiratory phase can be triggered by the patient as he or she makes an inspiratory effort. The term "assisted ventilation" is sometimes given to this mode of operation. Many constant-pressure ventilators have this capability. These ventilators are sometimes useful in the treatment of patients who are recovering from respiratory failure and who are being weaned from a period of controlled ventilation.

---

## ▶ Patterns of Ventilation

### Intermittent Positive Pressure Ventilation

Sometimes called intermittent positive pressure breathing (IPPB), intermittent positive pressure ventilation (IPPV) is the common pattern in which the lung is expanded by the application of positive pressure to the airway and is allowed to deflate passively to functional residual capacity (FRC). With modern ventilators, the main variables that can be controlled include the tidal volume, respiratory frequency, duration of inspiration versus expiration, the inspiratory flow rate, and the inspired oxygen concentration.

In patients with airway obstruction, there is an advantage in prolonging the expiratory time so that regions of the lung with long time constants have time to empty. (See *Respiratory Physiology: The Essentials*, 9th ed., p. 174). This can be done by reducing the respiratory frequency and increasing the expiratory versus inspiratory time. On the other hand, a prolonged positive airway pressure may impede venous return to the thorax (see later in this chapter). Generally, a relatively low frequency and an expiratory time greater than inspiratory time are selected, but each patient requires individual attention.

### Positive End-Expiratory Pressure (PEEP)

In patients who have ARDS, considerable improvement in the arterial $P_{O_2}$ can often be obtained by maintaining a small positive airway pressure at the end of expiration. Values as low as 5 cm $H_2O$ are often beneficial, but pressures of 20 cm $H_2O$ or more are sometimes used. Special valves are available to provide the pressure. A secondary gain from positive end-expiratory pressure (PEEP) is that it may allow the inspired oxygen concentration to be decreased, thus lessening the risk of oxygen toxicity.

Several mechanisms are probably responsible for the increase in arterial $P_{O_2}$ resulting from PEEP. The positive pressure increases the FRC, which is typically small in these patients because of the increased elastic recoil of the lung. The low lung volume causes airway closure and intermittent ventilation (or none at all) of some areas, especially in the dependent regions (see Figure 3-4), and absorption atelectasis ensues (see Figure 9-4). PEEP tends to reverse these changes. Patients with edema in their airways also benefit, probably because the fluid is moved into small peripheral airways or alveoli, allowing some regions of the lung to be reventilated.

Figure 10-2 shows the effects of PEEP in a patient with ARDS. Note that the level of PEEP was progressively increased from 0 to 16 cm $H_2O$, and this caused the shunt to fall from 43.8 to 14.2% of the cardiac output. A small amount of blood flow to poorly ventilated alveoli remained. The increase in PEEP also caused the dead space to increase from 36.3 to 49.8% of the tidal volume. This can be explained by compression of the capillaries by the increased alveolar pressure and also the increase in volume of the lung and consequent increased radial traction on the airways, which increases their volume. This situation is discussed further below.

Occasionally, the addition of too much PEEP reduces rather than increases the arterial $P_{CO_2}$. Possible mechanisms include (1) a substantial fall in cardiac output, which reduces the $P_{O_2}$ of

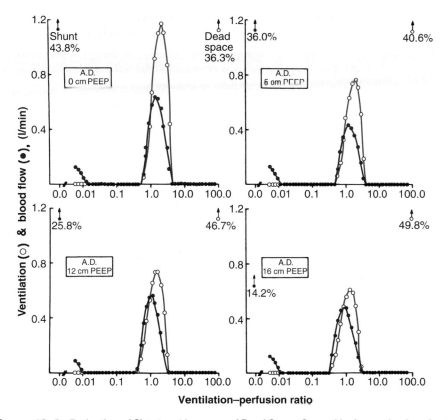

**Figure 10-2.** Reduction of Shunt and Increase of Dead Space Caused by Increasing Levels of PEEP In a Patient with Adult Respiratory Distress Syndrome (ARDS). Note that as the PEEP was progressively increased from 0 to 16 cm $H_2O$, the shunt decreased from 43.8 to 14.2% of the cardiac output, and the dead space increased from 36.3 to 49.8% of the tidal volume. (From Dantzker DR, Brook CJ, DeHart P, et al. Ventilation–perfusion distributions in the adult respiratory distress syndrome. *Am Rev Respir Dis* 1979;120:1039–1052.)

mixed venous blood and therefore the arterial $P_{O_2}$; (2) reduced ventilation of well-perfused regions (because of increasing dead space and ventilation to poorly perfused regions); and (3) diversion of blood flow away from ventilated to unventilated regions by the raised airway pressure. These deleterious effects of PEEP on the arterial $P_{O_2}$ are fortunately seldom seen.

PEEP tends to reduce cardiac output by impeding venous return to the thorax, especially if the circulating blood volume has been depleted by hemorrhage or shock. Accordingly, its value should not be gauged by its effect on the arterial $P_{O_2}$ alone but in terms of the total amount of oxygen delivered to the tissues. The product of the arterial oxygen concentration and the cardiac output is a useful index because changes in this alter the $P_{O_2}$ of mixed venous blood and therefore the $P_{O_2}$ of many tissues. Some physicians use the level of the $P_{O_2}$ in mixed venous blood as a guide to the optimal level of PEEP.

In some extremely ill patients, however, the $P_{O_2}$ of mixed venous blood can be misleading. Under some conditions, the application of PEEP causes a reduction in overall oxygen consumption of the patient. Although this raises the oxygen concentration and $P_{O_2}$ of mixed venous blood (see Equation 9.2), this is not beneficial to the patient. Apparently, the oxygen consumption falls because the perfusion of some tissues is so marginal that if their blood flow is further decreased, they are unable to take up oxygen and presumably slowly die.

> ## Positive End-Expiratory Pressure (PEEP)
>
> - Often valuable for raising the arterial $P_{O_2}$ in patients with respiratory failure.
> - Values of 5 to 20 cm $H_2O$ are commonly used.
> - May allow the inspired $O_2$ concentration to be reduced.
> - May reduce cardiac output by impeding venous return.
> - High levels of PEEP may damage pulmonary capillaries.

Another hazard of high levels of PEEP is damage to the pulmonary capillaries as a result of the high tension in the alveolar walls. The alveolar wall can be considered a string of capillaries. High levels of tension greatly increase the stresses on the capillary walls, causing disruption of the alveolar epithelium, capillary endothelium, or sometimes all layers of the wall. This is another example of "stress failure," which was discussed in Chapter 6 in relation to pulmonary edema caused by high capillary hydrostatic pressures.

## Continuous Positive Airway Pressure (CPAP)

Some patients who are being weaned from a ventilator breathe spontaneously but are still intubated. Such patients may benefit from a small positive pressure applied continuously to the airway by a valve system on the ventilator. The improvement in oxygenation results from the same mechanisms as for PEEP. A form of continuous positive airway pressure has been used successfully in the treatment of infant respiratory distress syndrome. Another form of CPAP is useful in treating sleep-disordered breathing caused by upper airway obstruction. Here the increased pressure is applied via a face mask that is worn by the patient all night.

## Intermittent Mandatory Ventilation (IMV)

Intermittent mandatory ventilation (IMV) is a modification of IPPV in which a large tidal volume is given at relatively infrequent intervals to an intubated patient who is breathing spontaneously. It is often combined with PEEP or CPAP. This pattern may be useful in weaning a patient from a ventilator and in preventing upper airway occlusion in obstructive sleep apnea by using nasal CPAP during the night.

## High-Frequency Ventilation

It is possible to maintain normal blood gases by very-high-frequency (approximately 20 cycles per second) positive pressure ventilation with low stroke volumes (50–100 ml). The lung is vibrated rather than expanded in the conventional way, and the transport of the gas occurs by a combination of diffusion and convection. One use is in patients in whom gas leaks from the lung via a bronchopleural fistula.

## ▶ Physiologic Effects of Mechanical Ventilation

## Reduction of Arterial $P_{CO_2}$

In general, mechanical ventilation is used to increase ventilation and improve pulmonary gas exchange in lungs where this is grossly impaired. The impairment may result either because the patient is not able to breathe spontaneously, as in neuromuscular disease, or because the lung itself is severely diseased, as in ARDS. Frequently, mechanical ventilation is begun because the arterial $P_{CO_2}$ is rising or already elevated, and it is usually effective at keeping arterial $P_{CO_2}$ in check or reducing it. In patients with airway obstruction in whom the oxygen cost of breathing is high, mechanical ventilation may appreciably reduce the oxygen uptake and $CO_2$ output, thus contributing to the fall in arterial $P_{CO_2}$.

The relationship between the arterial $P_{CO_2}$ and the alveolar ventilation in normal lungs is given by the alveolar ventilation equation:

$$P_{CO_2} = \frac{\dot{V}_{CO_2}}{\dot{V}_A} \cdot K,$$   (Eq. 10.1)

where K is a constant. In diseased lungs, the denominator $\dot{V}_A$ in this equation is less than the ventilation going to the alveoli because of alveolar dead space, that is, unperfused alveoli or those with high ventilation–perfusion ratios. For this reason, the denominator is sometimes referred to as the "effective alveolar ventilation."

Mechanical ventilation frequently increases both the alveolar and anatomic dead spaces. As a consequence, the effective alveolar ventilation is not increased as much as the total ventilation. This is particularly likely if high pressures are applied to the airway. This can be seen in the example shown in Figure 10-2. As the level of PEEP was increased from 0 to 16 cm $H_2O$ in this patient with ARDS, the dead space increased from 36.3 to 49.8%. In some patients, high levels of PEEP also result in the appearance of lung units with high ventilation–perfusion ratios that cause a shoulder to form on the right of the ventilation distribution curve. This did not occur in the example shown. Occasionally, a large physiologic dead space is seen with IPPV even in the absence of PEEP. An example is shown in Figure 8-3.

There are several reasons why positive pressure ventilation increases dead space. First, lung volume is usually raised, especially when PEEP is added, and the resulting radial traction on the airways increases the anatomic dead space. Next, the raised airway pressure tends to divert blood flow away from ventilated regions, thus causing areas of high ventilation–perfusion ratio or even unperfused areas (Figure 10-2). This is particularly likely to happen in the uppermost regions of the lung where the pulmonary artery pressure is relatively low because of the hydrostatic effect. (See *Respiratory Physiology: The Essentials*, 9th ed., p. 46). Indeed, if the pressure in the capillaries falls below airway pressure, the capillaries may collapse completely, resulting in unperfused lung (Figure 10-3). This collapse is encouraged by two factors: (1) the abnormally high airway pressure and (2) the reduced venous return and consequent hypoperfusion of the lung. The latter is particularly likely to occur if there is a reduced circulating blood volume (see later in this chapter).

The tendency for the arterial $P_{CO_2}$ to rise as a result of the increased dead space can be countered by resetting the ventilator to increase the total ventilation. Nevertheless, it is important to remember that an increase in mean airway pressure can cause a substantial rise in dead space, although the increased pressure may be necessary to combat the shunt and resulting hypoxemia (Figure 10-2).

In practice, many patients who are mechanically ventilated develop an abnormally low arterial $P_{CO_2}$ because they are overventilated. This results in a respiratory alkalosis that frequently coexists with a metabolic acidosis because of the hypoxemia and impaired peripheral circulation. An unduly low arterial $P_{CO_2}$ should be avoided because it reduces cerebral blood flow and therefore contributes to cerebral hypoxia.

Another hazard of overventilation of patients with $CO_2$ retention is a low serum potassium, which predisposes to abnormal heart rhythms. When $CO_2$ is retained, potassium moves out of the cells into the plasma and is excreted by the kidney. If the $P_{CO_2}$ is then rapidly reduced, the potassium moves back into the cells, thus depleting the plasma.

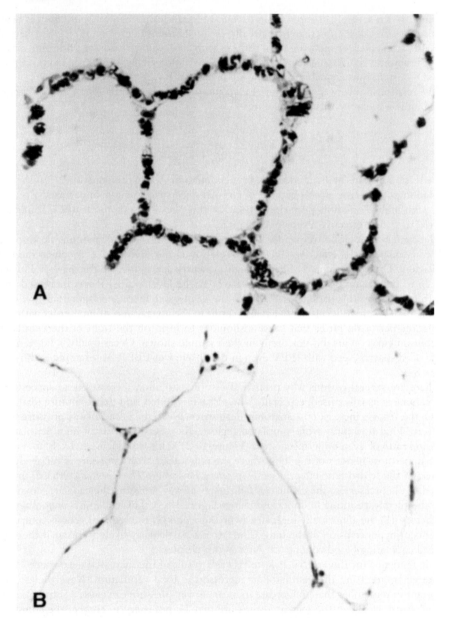

**Figure 10-3.** Effect of Raised Airway Pressure on the Histologic Appearance of Pulmonary **Capillaries. A.** Normal appearance. **B.** Collapse of capillaries when alveolar pressure is raised above capillary pressure. (From Glazier JB, Hughes JMB, Maloney JE, et al. Measurements of capillary dimensions and blood volume in rapidly frozen lungs. *J Appl Physiol* 1969;26:65–76.)

## Increase in Arterial $P_{O_2}$

In some patients with respiratory failure, for example, those with ARDS, the arterial $P_{CO_2}$ is not raised and the objective of mechanical ventilation is to increase the $P_{O_2}$. In practice, such patients are always ventilated with oxygen-enriched mixtures, and the combination is often effective in relieving the hypoxemia. The inspired oxygen concentration should ideally be sufficient to raise the arterial $P_{O_2}$ to at least 60 mm Hg, but unduly high inspired concentrations should be avoided because of the hazards of oxygen toxicity and atelectasis.

In some patients with severe forms of ARDS, IPPV with 100% $O_2$ is not successful in raising the arterial $P_{O_2}$ to 60 mm Hg. In these circumstances, the life-threatening hypoxemia of these patients can often be relieved by the addition of PEEP of 5 to 20 cm $H_2O$ (Figure 10-2). As noted earlier, this probably acts in several ways. The resulting increase in lung volume opens up atelectatic areas and reduces intermittent airway closure, particularly in the dependent regions. Also, edema fluid in the larger airways is moved peripherally, thus allowing some previously obstructed areas to be ventilated. As an example, the patient whose lung biopsy is shown in Figure 8-2 was put on 10 cm $H_2O$ PEEP on the day after the biopsy was taken. This resulted in a rise in arterial $P_{O_2}$ from 80 to 130 mm Hg during 80% oxygen breathing.

## Effects on Venous Return

Mechanical ventilation tends to impede the return of blood into the thorax and thus reduce the cardiac output. This is true for both positive pressure and negative pressure ventilation. In a supine, relaxed patient, the return of blood to the thorax depends on the difference between the peripheral venous pressure and the mean intrathoracic pressure. If the airway pressure is increased by a ventilator, mean intrathoracic pressure rises and venous return is impeded. Even if airway pressure remains atmospheric, as in a tank respirator, venous return tends to fall because the peripheral venous pressure is reduced by the negative pressure. Only with the cuirass respirator is venous return virtually unaffected.

The effects of positive pressure ventilation on venous return depend on the magnitude and duration of the inspiratory pressure, and particularly, on the addition of PEEP. The ideal pattern from this standpoint is a short inspiratory phase of relatively low pressure followed by a long expiratory phase and zero (or slightly negative) end-expiratory pressure. However, such a pattern encourages a low lung volume and consequent hypoxemia, and a compromise is generally necessary.

An important determinant of venous return is the magnitude of the circulating blood volume. If this is reduced, for example, by hemorrhage or shock, positive-pressure ventilation often causes a marked fall in cardiac output. Systemic hypotension may ensue. It is therefore important to correct any volume depletion by appropriate fluid replacement. The central venous pressure is often monitored as a guide to this but should be interpreted in the light of the increased airway pressure. Positive airway pressure itself raises central venous pressure. An additional factor often contributing to the fall in cardiac output during mechanical ventilation is hypocapnia caused by overventilation.

## Miscellaneous Hazards

*Mechanical problems* are a constant hazard. They include power failure, broken connections, and kinking of tubes. Apnea alarms are available to warn of these dangers, but skilled care by the intensive care team is essential.

*Pneumothorax* can occur, especially if PEEP and/or unusually large tidal volumes are used. *Interstitial emphysema* may develop if the lung is overdistended. The air escapes from ruptured alveoli, tracks along the perivascular and peribronchial interstitium (see Figure 6-1), and may enter the mediastinum and the subcutaneous tissue of the neck.

*Pulmonary infection* is a danger if the equipment is not scrupulously clean. Crusting of the large airways occurs unless the gas is efficiently humidified. *Cardiac arrhythmias* may be caused by rapid swings in pH and hypoxemia. There is also an increased incidence of *gastrointestinal bleeding* in these patients.

## KEY CONCEPTS

1. Mechanical ventilation has a major role in treating patients with respiratory failure, for example, in the intensive care unit. The ventilator is connected to the patient's airway via an endotracheal tube, or sometimes via a tracheostomy tube.

2. The commonest types of ventilators include constant-volume and constant-pressure ventilators. Tank ventilators are now seldom used except for patients with long-term neuromuscular disease.

3. The usual mode of ventilation is intermittent positive pressure ventilation (IPPV), and this is frequently combined with positive end-expiratory pressure (PEEP) in patients with the adult respiratory distress syndrome.

4. Mechanical ventilation, especially when used with an increased oxygen concentration and PEEP, typically increases the arterial $P_{O_2}$ and reduces the $P_{CO_2}$. However, it can reduce venous return and may cause a pneumothorax.

## QUESTIONS

1. Concerning endotracheal tubes:
   A. They are easily obstructed if the patient vomits.
   B. They are easily inserted by an untrained person.
   C. They facilitate the removal of retained secretions by suction.
   D. The cuff invariably damages the airway wall.
   E. They increase the anatomic dead space.

2. Constant-volume ventilators:
   A. Do not allow the respiratory frequency to be changed.
   B. Provide a nearly constant tidal volume even if lung compliance falls.
   C. Have a fixed ratio of inspiratory to expiratory time.
   D. Do not require electrical power.
   E. Are typically small and portable.

3. In the treatment of a patient with ARDS by mechanical ventilation, the addition of PEEP typically results in:
   A. Reduced arterial $P_{O_2}$.
   B. Reduced FRC.
   C. Increased shunt.
   D. Reduced physiologic dead space.
   E. Tendency to reduce venous return to the thorax.

4. A patient with paralyzed respiratory muscles but normal lungs is being treated by mechanical ventilation. In this patient the arterial $P_{CO_2}$ can be reduced without changing total ventilation by:
   A. Reducing the FRC.
   B. Increasing the tidal volume.
   C. Increasing the respiratory frequency.
   D. Reducing the resistance of the airways.
   E. Adding oxygen to the inspired gas.

5. Hazards of mechanical ventilation include:
   A. Centriacinar emphysema.
   B. Pulmonary edema.
   C. Pulmonary fibrosis.
   D. Pneumothorax.
   E. Anemia.

# Symbols, Units, and Normal Values

## ▶ SYMBOLS

### Primary

| | |
|---|---|
| C | Concentration of gas in blood |
| F | Fractional concentration in dry gas |
| P | Pressure or partial pressure |
| Q | Volume of blood |
| $\dot{Q}$ | Volume of blood per unit time |
| R | Respiratory exchange ratio |
| S | Saturation of hemoglobin with $O_2$ |
| V | Volume of gas |
| $\dot{V}$ | Volume of gas per unit time |

### Secondary Symbols for Gas Phase

| | |
|---|---|
| A | Alveolar |
| B | Barometric |
| D | Dead space |
| E | Expired |
| I | Inspired |
| L | Lung |
| T | Tidal |

### Secondary Symbols for Blood Phase

| | |
|---|---|
| a | arterial |
| c | capillary |
| c′ | end-capillary |
| i | ideal |
| v | venous |
| $\bar{v}$ | mixed venous |

### Examples

$O_2$ concentration in arterial blood $Ca_{O_2}$
Fractional concentration of $N_2$ in expired gas $Fe_{N_2}$
Partial pressure of $O_2$ in mixed venous blood $P\bar{v}_{O_2}$

## ► UNITS

Traditional metric units are used in this book. Pressures are given in mm Hg; the torr is an almost identical unit.

In Europe, SI (Système International) units are now commonly used. Most of them are familiar, but the kilopascal, the unit of pressure, is confusing at first. One kilopascal = 7.5 mm Hg (approximately).

### Conversion of Gas Volumes to BTPS

Lung volumes, including FEV and FVC, are conventionally expressed at body temperature (37°C), ambient pressure, and saturated with water vapor (BTPS). To convert volumes measured in a spirometer at ambient temperature (t), pressure, saturated (ATPS) to BTPS,

$$\frac{310}{273+t} \cdot \frac{P_B - P_{H_2O}(t)}{P_B - 47}$$

In practice, tables are available for this conversion.

The derivation of this equation and all the other equations is given in the companion volume (*Respiratory Physiology: The Essentials*, 9th ed., pp. 180–185).

## ► REFERENCE VALUES

## Reference Values for Lung Function Tests

Normal values depend on age, gender, height, weight, and ethnic origin. This is a complex subject; for a detailed discussion, see pages 445–513 of Cotes JE. *Lung Function*. 5th ed. Oxford: Blackwell, 1993. Reference values for some common tests are shown in Table A.1. There is evidence that people are becoming healthier and that lung function is improving.

| Table A.1 | Example of Reference Values for Common Pulmonary Function Tests in White Nonsmoking Adults in the United States | |
|---|---|---|
| | **Men** | **Women** |
| TLC (l) | 7.95 St* + 0.003 A† − 7.33 (0.79)‡ | 5.90 St − 4.54 (0.54) |
| FVC (l) | 7.74 St − 0.021 A − 7.75 (0.51) | 4.14 St − 0.023 A − 2.20 (0.44) |
| RV (l) | 2.16 St + 0.021 A − 2.84 (0.37) | 1.97 St + 0.020 A − 2.42 (0.38) |
| FRC (l) | 4.72 St + 0.009 A − 5.29 (0.72) | 3.60 St + 0.003 A − 3.18 (0.52) |
| RV/TLC (%) | 0.309 A + 14.1 (4.38) | 0.416 A + 14.35 (5.46) |
| $FEV_1$ (l) | 5.66 St − 0.023 A − 4.91 (0.41) | 2.68 St − 0.025 A − 0.38 (0.33) |
| $FEV_1$/FVC (%) | 110.2 − 13.1 St − 0.15 A (5.58) | 124.4 − 21.4 St − 0.15 A (6.75) |
| $FEF_{25-75\%}$ (l $s^{-1}$) | 5.79 St − 0.036 A − 4.52 (1.08) | 3.00 St − 0.031 A − 0.41 (0.85) |
| $MEF_{50\% FVC}$ (l $s^{-1}$) | 6.84 St − 0.037 A − 5.54 (1.29) | 3.21 St − 0.024 A − 0.44 (0.98) |
| $MEF_{25\% FVC}$ (l $s^{-1}$) | 3.10 St − 0.023 A − 2.48 (0.69) | 1.74 St − 0.025 A − 0.18 (0.66) |
| DI (ml $min^{-1}$ mm $Hg^{-1}$) | 16.4 St − 0.229 A + 12.9 (4.84) | 16.0 St − 0.111 A + 2.24 (3.95) |
| DI/$V_A$ | 10.09 − 2.24 St − 0.031 A (0.73) | 8.33 − 1.81 St − 0.016 A (0.80) |

*St is stature (height) (m).

†A is age (years).

‡Standard deviation is in parentheses.

From Cotes JE. *Lung Function*. 5th ed. Oxford, UK: Blackwell, 1993.

# Further Reading

Crystal RG, West JB, Weibel ER, Barnes PJ. *The Lung: Scientific Foundations*. 2nd ed. Philadelphia, PA: Lippincott-Raven, 1997.

Mason RJ, Courtney Broaddus V, Martin TR, King TE, Schraufnagel DE, Murray JF, Nadel JA. *Murray and Nadel's Textbook of Respiratory Medicine*. 5th ed. Philadelphia, PA: Saunders Elsevier, 2010.

Fishman AP (Editor-in-Chief). *Fishman's Pulmonary Diseases and Disorders*. 4th ed. New York, NY: McGraw-Hill, 2008.

Kumar V, Abbas AK, Fausto N, Aster J. *Robbins and Cotran Pathologic Basis of Disease*. Philadelphia, PA: Saunders/Elsevier, 2010.

# Answers to Chapter Questions

## Chapter 1

1. B is correct. An effective bronchodilator increases the $FEV_1$ and often the FVC. The other choices are incorrect. The test is easy to perform, the result is greatly affected by dynamic compression of the airways, the FEV is reduced in fibrosis but also in COPD, and the FEV decreases with age.

2. E is correct. Dynamic compression of the airways is the most important mechanism limiting maximum flow rate during most of a forced expiration. The other choices are incorrect. Turbulence in the trachea does occur but is not a limiting factor. The action of the diaphragm, contraction of intercostal muscles, and power of abdominal muscles could increase the expiratory effort, but during dynamic compression of the airways, flow is effort-independent.

3. A is correct. The $FEV_1$ in the patient with COPD is largely determined by dynamic compression of the airways during which the driving pressure is alveolar minus intrapleural pressure. This pressure difference is reduced if lung compliance is increased. The other choices are incorrect. Increase in the number of small airways, increased radial traction on the airways, and increased elastic recoil of the lung will all tend to increase the flow rate during dynamic compression. Hypertrophy of the diaphragm is not a factor because flow is effort-independent.

4. C is correct. In a patient with interstitial fibrosis, the $FEV_1$/FVC is increased because of the greater radial traction holding the airways open compared with the normal lung. The other choices are incorrect. Both the $FEV_1$ and FVC are decreased, but the expiratory flow rate when related to lung volume is increased, again because of the increased radial traction on the airways. Early in expiration, the flow rate depends on expiratory effort, but this is not increased in these patients.

5. A is correct. Fixed upper airway obstruction reduces both the inspiratory and expiratory flow rates. The other choices are incorrect. The response to bronchodilator drugs is best measured during expiration, and the inspiratory flow–volume curve is not useful for differentiating between chronic bronchitis and emphysema, detecting resistance in small airways, or detecting fatigue of the diaphragm.

6. B is correct. The slope of phase 3 is increased in chronic bronchitis because poorly ventilated units receive less oxygen during the inspiration, and also they tend to empty last. The other choices are incorrect. The single breath nitrogen test is abnormal in mild COPD, poorly ventilated units tend to empty last, in normal subjects the last expired gas comes from the upper part of the lung, and during the test the expiratory flow rate should be limited to $0.5 \, \mathrm{l \, s^{-1}}$.

7. C is correct. The closing volume is raised when there is an increase in resistance of the small, peripheral airways because they then close at an abnormally high volume. The other choices are incorrect. Closing volume increases with age, it is poorly reproducible, it is most informative in patients with relatively mild lung disease, and it is raised in mild COPD.

## Chapter 2

1. D is correct. An increased 2,3-DPG concentration allows more oxygen to be unloaded because it reduces the oxygen affinity of hemoglobin, that is, it shifts the dissociation curve to the right. All the other choices increase the oxygen affinity.

2. C is correct. The arterial $P_{CO_2}$ is inversely related to the alveolar ventilation. Since the normal arterial $P_{CO_2}$ is 40, only a 20% reduction in ventilation is necessary to raise the $P_{CO_2}$ to 50 mm Hg. However, as Figure 2-2 shows, this small reduction in ventilation is not sufficient to reduce the arterial $P_{O_2}$ to 50 mm Hg or the oxygen saturation to 50%. There will be a small rise in plasma bicarbonate concentration, but since the normal value is 24, the end result will be <50. Base excess will not be altered.

3. C is correct. Doubling the $P_{CO_2}$ from 40 to 80 mm Hg causes a fall in pH of approximately 0.2 units (see page 18).

4. A is correct. Since the $P_{CO_2}$ is raised and the pH is reduced, there is a respiratory acidosis. However, the pH of 7.20 is too low to be explained by the $P_{CO_2}$ of 50 mm Hg, and so there must be a concomitant metabolic acidosis. This is common after surgery because a reduced blood flow and the resulting tissue hypoxia in some areas results in the production of lactic acid.

5. D is correct. The only mechanism of hypoxemia that prevents the arterial $P_{O_2}$ from reaching the expected level if 100% oxygen is inspired is shunt. In all the other mechanisms, the $P_{O_2}$ will rise to the expected level although this may take a long time with severe ventilation–perfusion inequality.

6. C is correct. CPAP is often the best treatment. The other choices are incorrect. The condition is common; many but not all patients are obese; sleep apnea is believed to be a factor in some patients with systemic hypertension, but treatment by CPAP reduces this; and snoring is common in sleep apnea.

7. B is correct. Breathing oxygen reduces the measured diffusing capacity for carbon monoxide because it reduces the rate of combination of CO with hemoglobin. The other choices are incorrect. The diffusing capacity is reduced in pulmonary fibrosis because of the increased thickness of the blood–gas barrier. The diffusing capacity is decreased by pneumonectomy because the area of the blood–gas barrier is reduced. Diffusion limitation of oxygen transfer during exercise is much more likely to occur at high altitude than at sea level principally because the $P_{O_2}$ in the blood is so low and the oxygen dissociation curve is so steep in that region. The diffusing capacity is best measured with carbon monoxide because the transfer of this gas is diffusion-limited, not because it moves slowly across the blood–gas barrier. In fact, the rate of diffusion of CO across the barrier is not particularly slow.

8. E is correct. Exercise at high altitude is one of the few situations where oxygen transfer is diffusion-limited in the normal lung. In none of the other four choices is gas transfer limited by diffusion, and therefore, doubling the diffusing capacity will have no effect.

9. E is correct. The reduced pH indicates an acidosis, but the fact that the $P_{CO_2}$ is reduced means that this cannot be respiratory. Furthermore, the bicarbonate concentration of 25 mmol $l^{-1}$ is normal or slightly high, and this rules out a metabolic acidosis. Therefore, there must be a laboratory error.

10. E is correct. The low pH indicates an acidosis and the fact that the $P_{CO_2}$ is low means that this must be metabolic. The other choices are incorrect. A is wrong because there is an acidosis not an alkalosis. B requires a simple calculation. Since the patient is breathing air, the inspired $P_{O_2}$ is about 150. Using the alveolar gas equation, the alveolar $P_{O_2}$ is therefore about 150-32/0.8, that is, about 110. Since the arterial $P_{O_2}$

is 70, the alveolar–arterial $P_{CO_2}$ difference is about 40, which is abnormal. C is incorrect because an arterial $P_{O_2}$ of 70 gives an $O_2$ saturation of much more than 70%. Recall that normal mixed venous blood has a $P_{O_2}$ of about 40 mm Hg and a saturation of about 75%. D is incorrect because the $P_{O_2}$ in a vein would be much <70 mm Hg.

## Chapter 3

1. D is correct. The FRC is the volume at which the elastic recoil of the lung and that of the chest wall balance each other. The other choices are incorrect. The FRC cannot be measured with a simple spirometer because it includes the residual volume. In patients with lung disease, the FRC measured by plethysmography is often larger than that measured by helium dilution because some lung units are behind obstructed airways and do not communicate with the mouth. The FRC is typically increased during an asthma attack, and the FRC rises with advancing age.

2. B is correct. $\beta_2$-agonists reduce airway resistance in asthma and indeed are some of the most valuable medications. The other choices are incorrect. Airway resistance is decreased at high lung volumes. Destruction of alveolar walls does not typically occur in asthma. Airway resistance is increased by obstructions in the airways, for example, retained secretions. Airway resistance is also increased by hypertrophy of bronchial smooth muscle, so we can expect loss of some of the muscle to decrease resistance.

3. A is correct. A patient with mitral stenosis tends to have a reduced cardiac output and therefore impaired perfusion of skeletal muscle at a relatively low level of exercise. The result will be an increased blood lactate level, which stimulates ventilation, and therefore, washes out $CO_2$ and causes the respiratory exchange ratio to rise about 1. The other choices are incorrect. The high respiratory exchange ratio is caused by an abnormally high ventilation, cardiac output is abnormally low, and lung compliance and diffusing capacity are not relevant.

4. D is correct. The alveoli at the top of the lungs are larger than those at the base because the lung tissue is distorted by its weight (see Figure 3-4). All the other choices are incorrect because they refer to variables that are reduced at the apex of the lung.

5. B is correct. Alveolar ventilation can increase 10-fold or more. All the other choices increase much less.

## Chapter 4

1. B is correct. Centriacinar emphysema initially occurs in the upper part of the lung see Figure 4-5A. The other choices are incorrect. The emphysema caused by $\alpha_1$-antitrypsin deficiency often preferentially affects the base of the lung. The other choices do not have a typical regional distribution.

2. C is correct. There is evidence that released neutrophil elastase attacks the elastin and collagen in the lung. The release of the elastase is apparently increased by cigarette smoke. The other choices are incorrect. Increased alveolar pressure is usually associated with an increased intrapleural pressure and does not damage the capillaries. Cigarette smoking stimulates bronchial mucous glands, but that is the pathogenesis of bronchitis, not of emphysema. Exercise and hyperventilation do not play a role in the pathogenesis of emphysema.

3. B is correct. The emphysema of $\alpha_1$-antitrypsin deficiency occurs at a relatively early age. The other choices are incorrect. $\alpha_1$-Antitrypsin deficiency does not cause bronchitis, it is not due to childhood infections, it is uncommon or absent in heterozygotes for the Z gene, and, if anything, it is most marked in the lower regions of the lung.

4. C is correct. Patients with a type A presentation tend to have large increase in lung compliance. The other choices are incorrect. These patients have less cough productive of sputum, larger lung volumes, less hypoxemia, and a lesser tendency to develop cor pulmonale. Some people might question whether C is always correct, but the other options are clearly incorrect so C is the best answer.

5. E is correct. All the features of a forced expiration listed in A through D are likely to be abnormal in a patient with severe bronchitis and emphysema.

6. C is correct. By far the commonest mechanism of hypoxemia in patients with COPD is ventilation–perfusion inequality. All the other choices are incorrect. Hypoventilation, diffusion impairment, and shunt typically do not occur. Choice E, abnormal hemoglobin, is irrelevant.

7. E is correct. The FRC often falls when a patient with asthma is treated with a bronchodilator. However, more important is that all the other options are clearly incorrect. All these measurements from a forced expiration typically increase following administration of a bronchodilator.

8. D is correct. β-Adrenergic agonists in asthma reduce airway inflammation and airway resistance. The other choices are incorrect. $\beta_2$-selective agonists are preferred to β1. The mechanism or relaxation of airway smooth muscle is by increasing the concentration of adenyl cyclase, which then increases the concentration of intracellular cAMP. The bronchodilators are given by inhalation.

## Chapter 5

1. D is correct. The type II alveolar epithelial cell secretes surfactant (or its precursor). The other choices are incorrect. The cell does not provide most of the structural support for the normal alveolar wall. This is done by the type I alveolar epithelial cell. The type II cells can multiply, whereas the type I cells cannot. When a type I cell is damaged, it is replaced by a type II cell. These cells are also very metabolically active.

2. A is correct. In diffuse interstitial pulmonary fibrosis, there is initially infiltration of the alveolar wall with lymphocytes and plasma cells. However, breakdown of alveolar walls is not a feature, and mucous gland hypertrophy in the bronchi and mucous plugging of airways do not occur. The volume of the pulmonary capillary bed is typically reduced.

3. D is correct. Dyspnea especially on exercise is a prominent feature of diffuse interstitial pulmonary fibrosis. The other choices are incorrect. There is often a dry unproductive cough, but this is not associated with copious sputum. Hemoptysis and rhonchi do not occur. The diaphragms are typically raised because of the increased lung elastic recoil and the resulting small lungs.

4. C is correct. Because of the increased radial traction on the airways, the $FEV_1/FVC$ percentage is typically increased. However, the $FEV_1$, FVC, and TLC are reduced. Airway resistance when related to lung volume is also reduced.

5. A is correct. The arterial $P_{O_2}$ of a patient with diffuse interstitial pulmonary fibrosis typically falls during exercise. The other choices are incorrect. The hypoxemia is chiefly caused by ventilation–perfusion inequality, not by diffusion impairment, though this can contribute to the hypoxemia during exercise. The diffusing capacity typically increases little on exercise. Carbon dioxide retention is not a feature. The hypoxemia worsens during exercise and is typically associated with an abnormally small increase in cardiac output.

6. D is correct. The increased radial traction on the airways explains the higher flow rate in relation to lung volume compared with a normal subject. The other choices are incorrect.

The high flow rate is not related to the mechanical advantage of the expiratory muscles, the airways have a larger diameter if anything, and dynamic compression of the airways is less likely than in a normal subject. Airway resistance is decreased.

7. D is correct. The diffusing capacity for carbon monoxide in a patient with diffuse interstitial lung disease is reduced in part because of a smaller capillary blood volume although another important factor is the thickening of the blood–gas barrier. The other choices are incorrect. The diffusing capacity is reduced, it shows an abnormally small increase during exercise, and, as indicated above, it is affected by the thickening of the blood–gas barrier. The diffusing capacity also falls relatively early in the disease, and indeed this may be a useful diagnostic pointer.

8. C is correct. A tension pneumothorax is a medical emergency and can be relieved by inserting a needle through the chest wall into the pneumothorax cavity. The other choices are incorrect. A pneumothorax increases the volume of the chest wall on the affected side and results in a reduced blood flow in the affected lung. Spontaneous pneumothorax is relatively common in young men and causes a reduction in the FVC.

## Chapter 6

1. C is correct. If the colloid osmotic pressure of the blood is reduced, there is less of a tendency for fluid to move into the capillaries. The other choices are incorrect. The permeability of the alveolar epithelial cells is not relevant to fluid movement between the capillary lumen and the interstitium of the alveolar wall. A reduced capillary hydrostatic pressure, an increased hydrostatic pressure in the interstitial space, and a reduced colloid osmotic pressure of the interstitial fluid will all tend to move fluid from the interstitium into the capillary lumen.

2. A is correct. In early interstitial edema, fluid moves from the capillary lumen into the interstitium of the thick side of the capillary wall. There is no movement of fluid into the thin side. The other choices are incorrect. The alveolar epithelium has a very low permeability for water, the strength of the barrier on the thin side is mainly attributable to the type IV collagen in the extracellular matrix, a small amount of protein normally crosses the capillary endothelium, and water is actively transported out of the alveolar spaces by alveolar epithelial cells.

3. E is correct. In early interstitial edema, cuffs of fluid collect around the small pulmonary arteries and veins. The other choices are incorrect. As stated in the answer to Question 2 above, fluid from the capillary lumen does not enter the thin side of the blood–gas barrier. In the early stages of pulmonary edema there is an increase in lung lymph flow. However, fluid does not enter the alveoli in interstitial edema. In early interstitial edema the hydrostatic pressure in the interstitium rises as fluid enters it, and this tends to inhibit further movement of fluid from the capillary lumen to the interstitium.

4. A is correct. Interstitial pulmonary edema is difficult to detect, but short, linear, horizontal markings near the pleural surface known as "septal lines" can be seen on a chest radiograph. The other choices are incorrect. Lung compliance falls, lymph flow from the lung increases, there is little if any impairment of gas exchange and certainly no severe hypoxemia, and fluffy shadowing occurs on the chest radiograph in alveolar edema but not interstitial edema.

5. D is correct. Positive pressure ventilation tends to move the fluid from the larger airways into the peripheral air spaces. The other choices are incorrect. Carbon dioxide retention is not typically seen, the fluid-filled alveoli become smaller because of surface tension effects, some red blood cells are always seen in alveolar edema fluid, and there is prominent shadowing on the chest radiograph.

6. E is correct. Hypoxic pulmonary vasoconstriction increases the pulmonary artery pressure, but it is now believed that the constriction is uneven so that some capillaries are exposed to the high pressure. This damages their walls, and the result is a high-permeability type of edema. The other choices are incorrect. The best evidence is that hypoxia does not itself increase capillary permeability although this was controversial at one time. Pulmonary venous pressure is not generally increased. Diuretics are not indicated, but the patient should descend as quickly as possible. Dyspnea is a prominent feature.

7. C is correct. Blood passing through regions of the lung with alveolar edema consti-tutes a shunt, and therefore there is hypoxemia while breathing 100% oxygen. The other choices are incorrect. Lung compliance is reduced, airway resistance is increased because some airways are blocked with fluid, respiration is typically shallow and rapid, but the edema does not cause chest pain.

8. D is correct. The use of oral contraceptives is associated with an increased risk of venous thrombosis. The other choices are incorrect. Overtransfusion with saline dilutes the blood and, if anything, reduces the tendency to thrombosis. Movement of the legs such as walking or leg exercise reduces the risk, as does anemia.

9. B is correct. The embolized areas do not eliminate $CO_2$, and therefore, the physiologic dead space is increased. The other choices are incorrect. $CO_2$ retention is not typical; pulmonary hypertension, not hypotension, occurs; rhonchi do not typically occur; car-diac output often falls.

10. A is correct. Long-standing COPD is associated with pulmonary hypertension, which increases the afterload of the right heart and can result in cor pulmonale. The other choices are incorrect. A reduced cardiac output is not always seen, cor pulmonale can also occur with severe diffuse interstitial pulmonary fibrosis, and the clinical signs typi-cally include neck vein engorgement, dependent edema, and a palpable liver.

## Chapter 7

1. D is correct. The most abundant pollutant in the atmosphere is carbon monoxide largely as a product of internal combustion engines. The other choices are incorrect. Hydrocar-bons, sulfur oxides, nitrogen oxides, and ozone are all important pollutants but occur in smaller concentrations.

2. D is correct. Nitrogen oxides in smog cause inflammation of the upper respiratory tract and are probably a factor in the development of chronic bronchitis. The other choices are incorrect. Ozone is not mainly produced by automobile engines but by the action of sunlight on hydrocarbons and nitrogen oxides in the atmosphere. The main cause of sulfur oxides is burning fossil fuel that contains sulfur. Scrubbing fuel gases is effective in removing particles but is expensive.

3. B is correct. Heavy cigarette smokers can have up to 10% of their hemoglobin bound to carbon monoxide, and there is evidence that this can impair cognitive skills. The other choices are incorrect. Inhaled smoke contains substantial amounts of carbon monoxide. Nicotine is highly addictive. Smoking is an important risk factor in coronary heart dis-ease, and the concentration of pollutants in inhaled cigarette smoke is typically higher than that in smog.

4. B is correct. Medium-sized particles frequently deposit in the region of the terminal and respiratory bronchioles by the process of sedimentation, and this is one reason why early airway disease occurs in these areas. The other choices are incorrect. The nose effectively filters out most particles larger than 5 μm in diameter, astronauts in space are in microgravity so that deposition by sedimentation does not occur, particles

of 0.5 µm diameter diffuse very much more slowly than gas molecules, and most parti-cles larger than 10 µm are captured in the nose and upper airways and never reach the lung.

5. E is correct. If a miner breathes through his nose, most of the larger particles will be trapped there. The other choices are incorrect. Coughing can help to remove particles but does not prevent their deposition. Exercise increases pulmonary ventilation and therefore increases deposition. Very small dust particles are deposited by sedimentation or diffusion, and rapid deep breathing increases deposition.

6. E is correct. The mucous film is altered in some diseases such as asthma, where it becomes tenacious and difficult for the cilia to move. The other choices are incorrect. Although goblet cells in the airway epithelium produce some mucus, most of it comes from the seromucous glands in the airway wall. Trapped particles move much more rapidly in the trachea than in the peripheral airways. Normal clearance is complete in about a day or so, and cilia typically beat around 20 times per second.

7. C is correct. In pneumonia, the lung affected by the disease is not ventilated, and if it is perfused, the resulting shunt can cause hypoxemia. The other choices are incorrect. Many patients with pneumonia recover with no residual pathology in the lung, the disease may cause pleuritic pain, and fever and cough often occur.

8. D is correct. Small-cell bronchial carcinomas are very common. The other choices are incorrect. The disease is more common in males; the carcinogenic agents in cigarette smoke, loosely described as tars, have not been fully identified; pulmonary function tests are not useful in the early detection of the disease, and some early carcinomas are not vis-ible on the chest radiograph.

9. E is correct. The responsible genetic defect has been identified, although successful gene therapy is not yet available. The other choices are incorrect. The disease also occurs in the pancreas; it was rare for affected children to reach the age of 20, but this is no longer the case because of improvements in supportive therapy. Finger clubbing is common, and the change in the composition of the sweat is a valuable diagnostic test.

# Chapter 8

1. B is correct. Patients with severe COPD and $CO_2$ retention (this patient's $P_{CO_2}$ was 50 mm Hg) often have their ventilation partly driven by the low arterial $P_{O_2}$. If they are treated with 100% oxygen, this drive to ventilation is removed, and they may decrease their ventilation with a corresponding increase in $P_{CO_2}$. The other choices are incor-rect. Administering oxygen does not increase airway resistance or depress cardiac output. Choices D and E are irrelevant.

2. B is correct. An exacerbation of a chest infection in a patient with respiratory failure can cause an increase in arterial $P_{CO_2}$ and therefore respiratory acidosis. The other choices are incorrect. Mechanical ventilation and administration of antibiotics will reduce the tendency to $CO_2$ retention. Renal retention of bicarbonate will reduce the acidosis by metabolic compensation.

3. D is correct. A patient with ARDS typically has severe hypoxemia caused by extensive ventilation–perfusion inequality, including blood flow through unventilated lung (shunt). The other choices are incorrect. Lung compliance and FRC are typically decreased, and a large shunt often occurs. The chest radiograph is markedly abnormal.

4. B is correct. The pathogenesis is insufficient pulmonary surfactant, and the result is patchy edema and atelectasis. The other choices are incorrect. There is inadequate pulmonary surfactant, and there is typically severe hypoxemia and a large shunt. The condition is most common in prematurely born children.

**5.** B is correct. An acute exacerbation of bronchitis in a patient with severe COPD typically causes worsening of the ventilation–perfusion relationships. The other choices are incorrect. The bronchitis increases the work of breathing, the arterial pH typically falls because of the respiratory acidosis, and an increase in the alveolar–arterial $P_{O_2}$ difference is usual. Mechanical ventilation may improve the gas exchange of such a patient, but often the decision whether to use it is difficult. A danger is that the patient may become ventilator-dependent.

## Chapter 9

**1.** E is correct. Fifty percent oxygen raises the inspired $P_{O_2}$ to about 350 mm Hg from its normal value of about 150 mm Hg. Therefore, if the $P_{CO_2}$ does not change, we can expect the arterial $P_{O_2}$ to rise by approximately 200 mm Hg.

**2.** D is correct. The arterial $P_{O_2}$ will rise because of the oxygen dissolved in the nonshunted blood. However, it cannot possibly rise to 600 mm Hg because of the shunt. Therefore, the only possible correct choices are C and D. Figure 9-3 and the accompanying text shows that the increase will be more than 10 mm Hg. However, choosing between C and D is challenging.

**3.** B is correct. The presence of carbon monoxide in blood increases its oxygen affinity. The other choices are incorrect. A patient with CO poisoning may have a normal arterial $P_{O_2}$, but this will not be increased, and even if it was, this would not affect the $P_{50}$. The other choices all cause an increase in the $P_{50}$ of the blood.

**4.** C is correct. The inspired oxygen concentration with nasal cannulas can change greatly depending on the pattern of breathing and whether the patient is partly breathing through his mouth. The other choices are incorrect. Most patients find cannulas more comfortable than masks, inspired oxygen concentrations about 25% can be obtained, there is no interference with the patient talking, and in most patients the $P_{CO_2}$ does not tend to rise. Although this could happen in a patient with respiratory failure whose respiratory drive comes partly from the arterial hypoxemia, the increase in arterial $P_{O_2}$ is usually not sufficient for this to occur.

**5.** E is correct. The solubility of oxygen is 0.003 ml 100 ml blood$^{-1}$ mm Hg$^{-1}$. A pressure of 3 atmospheres is equivalent to 2280 mm Hg so that with an inspired concentration of 100% we can expect the inspired $P_{O_2}$ to rise to more than 2000 mm Hg. Therefore, the amount of dissolved oxygen will be approximately 6 ml 100 ml$^{-1}$.

**6.** D is correct. Studies on primates that have been exposed to 100% oxygen for many hours show the initial pathological changes in the capillary endothelial cells. A rule of thumb is that to prevent damage to the lung, 50% oxygen should not be given for more than 48 hours.

**7.** C is correct. When high concentrations of oxygen are administered, lung units with low ventilation–perfusion ratios may deliver oxygen into the blood faster than it is entering them by ventilation. The units therefore collapse. The other choices are incorrect. Pulmonary surfactant is not affected. Oxygen toxicity can cause alveolar edema, but this is not the mechanism of the collapse. Interstitial edema may occur around small airways, but this is not the mechanism, nor is any inflammatory changes in small airways, if in fact this does occur.

## Chapter 10

**1.** C is correct. Suction tubes can easily be inserted through an endotracheal tube in order to remove retained secretions. The other choices are incorrect. Vomitus does not obstruct an endotracheal tube because the tube is sealed in the airway with a cuff. Inserting an endotracheal tube requires training, particularly for negotiating the larynx, which requires local anesthesia. With some of the earlier endotracheal tubes, the cuff damaged the wall because of pressure, but this is now much less of a problem. The tube does not increase the anatomic dead space; in fact, it may reduce it.

2. B is correct. Constant-volume ventilators maintain a nearly constant tidal volume even if the compliance of the lung becomes less. The other choices are incorrect. Modern constant-volume ventilators allow the respiratory frequency to be changed and also the ratio of inspiratory to expiratory time. They require electrical power and are typically large machines that are not portable.

3. E is correct. Positive end-expiratory pressure (PEEP) tends to reduce venous return to the thorax because it increases intrathoracic pressure. The other choices are incorrect. Typically, the addition of PEEP increases the arterial $P_{O_2}$, increases the FRC, reduces shunt, but increases physiologic dead space.

4. B is correct. If the total ventilation is kept constant, the alveolar ventilation can be raised by increasing the tidal volume. This raises the ratio of alveolar ventilation to total ventilation, but of course reduces the respiratory frequency. The other choices are incorrect. Reducing the FRC will not directly affect ventilation, although it may result in atelectatic areas. Increasing the respiratory frequency necessarily means lowering the tidal volume, and thus reducing the ratio of alveolar ventilation to total ventilation. Reducing the resistance of the airways, if that can be done, will not change alveolar ventilation. Finally, adding oxygen to the inspired gas also does not change alveolar ventilation, although frequently this is initially confusing for students.

5. D is correct. Occasionally, mechanical ventilation will result in a pneumothorax, possibly because of overinflation of some regions of the lung, causing rupture of a bleb or some other part of the lung tissue. All the other choices are incorrect and are basically irrelevant to mechanical ventilation.

# Index

Note: Page numbers followed by italics indicate figures; pages followed by t indicate tables.